WHITE CELLS IN INFLAMMATION

Selected from communications presented
at meetings of The Inflammation Research Association

WHITE CELLS IN INFLAMMATION

Edited by

C. GORDON VAN ARMAN, Ph.D.

Merck Institute for Therapeutic Research
West Point, Pennsylvania

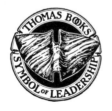

CHARLES C THOMAS • PUBLISHER

Springfield • Illinois • U.S.A.

Published and Distributed Throughout the World by
CHARLES C THOMAS • PUBLISHER
Bannerstone House
301-327 East Lawrence Avenue, Springfield, Illinois, U.S.A.

© *1974, by* CHARLES C THOMAS • PUBLISHER
ISBN 0-398-03120-7
Library of Congress Catalog Card Number: 74-896

*With THOMAS BOOKS careful attention is given to all details of
manufacturing and design. It is the Publisher's desire to present
books that are satisfactory as to their physical qualities and artistic
possibilities and appropriate for their particular use. THOMAS
BOOKS will be true to those laws of quality that assure a good
name and good will.*

Library of Congress Cataloging in Publication Data

Inflammation Research Association.
 White cells in inflammation.

 "Selected from communications presented at meetings of
the Inflammation Research Association."
 1. Inflammation—Congresses. 2. Leucocytes—
Congresses. I. Van Arman, C. Gordon, ed. II. Title.
[DNLM: 1. Inflammation—Congresses. 2. Leukocytes—
Congresses. WH200 W583 1974]
RB131.I54 1974 616'.047 74-896
ISBN 0-398-03120-7

Printed in the United States of America
CC-II

iv

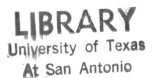

CONTRIBUTORS

A. W. Macklin, Ph.D.: Group Leader, Department of Toxicology and Experimental Pathology, Wellcome Research Laboratories, Burroughs Wellcome Company (U.S.A.) Incorporated, Research Triangle Park, North Carolina.

Michael E. Norman, M.D.: Instructor, Department of Pediatrics, University of Pennsylvania School of Medicine, Philadelphia; Acting Director, Laboratory of Clinical Immunology, Children's Hospital, Philadelphia, Pennsylvania.

H. Ralph Schumacher, M.D.: Director, Arthritis Research, Veterans Administration Hospital, Philadelphia, Pennsylvania; Associate Professor, Arthritis Section, Department of Medicine, Hospital of the University of Pennsylvania, Philadelphia, Pennsylvania.

J. L. Selph, B.S.: Research Assistant, Department of Pharmacology, Wellcome Research Laboratories, Burroughs Wellcome Company (U.S.A.) Incorporated, Research Triangle Park, North Carolina.

J. Bryan Smith, Ph.D.: Instructor in Pharmacology, Cardeza Foundation and Department of Pharmacology, Thomas Jefferson Medical School, Philadelphia, Pennsylvania.

W. G. Spector, M.D.: Director and Professor of Pathology, St. Bartholomew's Hospital Medical College, London, England

Robert S. Speirs, Ph.D.: Professor of Anatomy, College of Medicine, Downstate Medical Center, State University of New York, Brooklyn, New York.

Elizabeth E. Speirs: Research Assistant, Department of Anatomy, College of Medicine, Downstate Medical Center, State University of New York, Brooklyn, New York.

J. F. Truax, B.S.: Research Assistant, Department of Pharmacology, Wellcome Research Laboratories, Burroughs Wellcome Company (U.S.A.) Incorporated, Research Triangle Park, North Carolina.

Ralph Vinegar, Ph.D.: Senior Research Pharmacologist, Wellcome Research Laboratories, Burroughs Wellcome Company (U.S.A.) Incorporated, Research Triangle Park, North Carolina.

D. A. Willoughby, M.D.: Professor of Experimental Pathology, St. Bartholomew's Hospital Medical College, London, England.

PREFACE

The Inflammation Research Association arose spontaneously from a lively discussion after a session at the meetings of the Federation of American Societies for Experimental Biology in April 1970. It is a loose, informal group of research workers (not planners or organizers, but active workers in laboratories) who meet several times a year to talk about inflammatory diseases from the laboratory point of view. It is a group of enthusiasts. There is no reason other than pure scientific enthusiasm for any of them to come to any of the meetings; there is no prestige connected with the association, there are no membership lists, no elected officers, no journal, no dues—and we want to keep it that way. Dr. R. I. Takesue, M. E. Rosenthale, and C. G. Van Arman and Mrs. Mary Lee Graeme have done the necessary chores so far.

When we asked twenty-eight pharmaceutical companies for small contributions, they all helped underwrite the expenses of the fledgling association. This little volume expresses our thanks to Abbott Laboratories; Ayerst Research Laboratories; Bristol Laboratories; Burroughs-Wellcome Company; Ciba-Geigy Pharmaceuticals; Endo Laboratories; American Hoechst Corporation; Hoffmann-La Roche; Lederle Laboratories; Mead-Johnson; McNeil Laboratories; Merck Sharp and Dohme; Merrell-National Laboratories; Norwich Pharmacal Company; Ortho Pharmaceutical Corporation; Chas. Pfizer and Company; A. H. Robins Company; Wm. H. Rorer; Sandoz Pharmaceuticals; Schering Corporation; Smith Kline and French Laboratories; E. R. Squibb and Sons; Sterling-Winthrop Research Laboratories; Upjohn Company; Vick Divisions Research; Wallace Laboratories; Warner-Lambert Research Institute; and Wyeth Laboratories.

Most of our meetings have been held at the New York Academy of Sciences. In 1972, however, at the Thomas Jefferson Medical School in Philadelphia, we held one meeting jointly with the members of the Philadelphia Physiological Society; certain material in this volume was presented at that meeting. We thank those scientific descendants of Benjamin Franklin, especially Professor Marion Siegman, for their cordial hospitality on that occasion and look forward to future joint meetings of the two groups.

C. GORDON VAN ARMAN

INTRODUCTION

In 1882, Cohnheim showed that, in the web of the frog's foot, or in the frog's tongue, white corpuscles emigrated from the blood vessels to irritated tissue. Since then, the concept has been gaining favor that the various forms of white cells of blood and tissues are important in inflammation. Many kinds of white cells are morphologically and functionally distinguishable. Not only must we take into account all the kinds of cells, but we must also bear in mind that they probably do not act singly; they seem to cooperate with each other very furtively and cleverly in order to perform their various deeds or misdeeds.

The white cells seem to be playing a game like "Button, button, who's got the button?" We ask certain questions. How, for example, do cells pass antibodies from one to another? Is complement necessary for such transfer? How, if at all, do platelets enter into the development of certain diseases—for example, adjuvant-induced arthritis in rats? Can we prevent acute inflammation by depleting an animal of certain leukocytes? Which ones? Hollander and his coworkers[1] have suggested that, in such chronic diseases as rheumatoid arthritis, certain interactions occur among cells; but how can we test this hypothesis at its several critical points?

Various diseases have certain characteristics in common—fever, for instance; and we recognize that fever may have many causes; so also may swelling, pain, vasodilation, and loss of function of certain organs and organ-systems. We do not know, however, whether the pathways from one event to another, with inflammatory disease as the consequent manifestation, are similar at all, or whether there are only slight

---

[1] Hollander, J. L., McCarty, D. J., Astorga, G., and Castro-Murillo, E.: Studies on the pathogenesis of rheumatoid joint inflammation. I. The "R.A. cell" and a working hypothesis. *Annals Int Med, 62:* 271–291, 1965.

changes in the chain of events, causing one disease to appear rather than another. For such reasons, we have attempted no authoritative definition of the word *inflammation*.

At meetings of the Inflammation Research Association, many such questions are tossed into the air, like volley-balls, and freely knocked about. In this volume, several of the presentations have been collected in order to show various aspects of the general problem. Discoveries have recently appeared at an accelerating rate, so that it is quite possible that by the time this volume appears, certain questions may be much better answered than at this writing. Some of the material presented herein may soon be outdated—but if so, we will be well pleased.

CONTENTS

WHITE CELLS IN INFLAMMATION

CHAPTER I

PLATELETS AND

PERMEABILITY FACTORS

J. B. SMITH

INTRODUCTION

HUMAN PLATELETS ARE RELEASED from megakaryocytes in bone marrow and circulate in the blood stream for about ten days. There is little doubt about their major function, for it has been clearly shown that intact platelets must be present in the circulation in order to maintain hemostasis. That platelets may have other functions as well is indicated by less clear evidence. As a result of the clinical observation that thrombocytopenia is often accompanied by spontaneous hemorrhages and petechiae (for review, see Marcus and Zucker, 1965), some scientists speculate that platelets are necessary to preserve the integrity of the vascular endothelium. Others speculate that platelets play a part in inflammatory reactions in the vasculature. Platelets accumulate in blood vessels adjacent to areas of inflammation (Cotran, 1965) and may contribute to the inflammatory response by releasing intracellular constituents which increase vascular permeability (Mustard, Movat, MacMorine, and Senyi, 1965). In the following pages, the current knowledge of platelet permeability factors is reviewed and evidence provided which supports the hypothesis that one of these factors is prostaglandin E_2. Furthermore, the finding that aspirin inhibits the production of platelet prostaglandins is discussed. First, however, some of the morphological characteristics of platelets are outlined.

3

PLATELET ULTRASTRUCTURE

Platelets are anucleate and the smallest cells in the blood. They have diameters of 2 to 3 μ. Microtubules are believed to play an important part in maintaining them in a disc-like shape. Platelets also contain a dense tubular system, which is sometimes found localized as a submarginal bundle adjacent to the microtubules; a system of vacuoles, which is probably continuous with the surface membrane; and mitochondria and glycogen (Hovig, 1968). The most striking intracellular feature of platelets, however, is the *alpha*-granules which have diameters of about 0.2 μ. It is generally considered that at least some of these granules are lysosomes. Acid proteases, such as acid phosphatase, β-glucuronidase, β-N-acetylglucosaminidase, and cathepsins, have been shown to be associated with isolated α-granules (Day, Holmsen, and Hovig, 1969). Another type of organelle, called the very dense granule because it is extremely osmophilic, is also seen inside many platelets. Much evidence has been cited to suggest strongly that this is the site of serotonin storage in the platelet (for review, see Pletscher, 1968). Apparently, this organelle also contains large amounts of ATP and ADP, which may in some way bind the serotonin. Only in the rabbit do platelets have a high concentration of histamine (Humphrey and Jaques, 1954).

PHAGOCYTOSIS

In 1938, L. M. Tocantins suggested that platelets may be important in body defense against foreign particles and microorganisms, but it was not until 1964 that research provided some foundation for that view. In that year, J. F. David-Ferreira noted that platelets exposed to thorotrast contained in their vacuoles, thorotrast particles and were therefore capable of phagocytosing particulate matter. Subsequent studies have shown that platelets can engulf ferritin, viruses, fat particles, carbon, antigen-antibody complexes, and polystyrene particles (see Mustard and Packham, 1968). The true importance of phagocytosis by platelets, however, remains to be ascertained.

RELEASE OF PERMEABILITY FACTORS

Appropriately, it was studies of phagocytosis by platelets that provided real evidence for the hypothesis that platelets play a part in inflammation. Mustard and his coworkers (1965) first demonstrated that, when platelets engulf antigen-antibody complexes or latex particles, they release factors which can increase vascular permeability. These researchers, finding, furthermore, that the factors are released by thrombin and collagen fragments of a size too great to be phagocytosed, also demonstrated that the factors can be released without phagocytosis. And, since the interaction of platelets with antigen-antibody complexes, thrombin, or collagen is accompanied by extensive degranulation, the researchers suggested that histamine, serotonin and lysosomal enzymes were the vascular-permeability factors released from platelets.

CHARACTERIZATION OF THE PERMEABILITY FACTORS

Extensive research on the properties of the permeability factors released from platelets was done by Packham, Nishizawa, and Mustard (1968). They found that the factors caused an accumulation of Evans blue or albumin-I^{131} at the site of their intradermal injection in guinea pigs, domestic pigs, and rabbits. This effect was suppressed by the prior administration of an antihistamine drug (mepyramine maleate or triprolidine hydrochloride). The factors could not be histamine, however, for they were released from pig or human platelets, which contain little or no histamine, nor could they be serotonin, for they were released from pig platelets depleted of serotonin by reserpine treatment. The factors were heat-stable and therefore unlikely to be one of the lysosomal enzymes known to be released from platelets. They also seemed to have molecular weights of less than 10,000. The factors, furthermore, caused contraction of the guinea-pig ileum, and, although this effect was partially inhibited by mepyramine maleate, it was unaffected by the antiserotonin drug, bromolysergic acid diethylamide. Finally, these workers showed that the release of the permeability factors from platelets was inhibited by aspirin or phenylbutazone. This finding, of course, lends support to the concept that the factors have some role in inflammation.

NATURE OF THE PERMEABILITY FACTORS

The properties Packham and his associates established in 1968 as characteristic of the permeability factors were inconsistent with the properties of any then fully accepted mediator of inflammation. The factors therefore presented an intriguing problem. They were of considerable importance; for, in order to develop more effective anti-inflammatory drugs, information was needed about all inflammatory mediators. Two lines of research, which may not be mutually exclusive, have since shed considerable light on the nature of the permeability factors.

Lipid

Prostaglandins are a family of polyunsaturated, hydroxyfatty acids with molecular weights of about 350. Certain members of this family, such as prostaglandin E_1 (PGE_1) or prostaglandin E_2 (PGE_2), contract the guinea-pig ileum (Bergström, Carlson, and Weeks, 1968). They therefore have an action in common with the platelet permeability factors. Furthermore, prostaglandins and platelet permeability factors have another action in common. As little as 1 ng of PGE_1 or PGE_2 injected into the skin of rats causes an increase in vascular permeability; and antihistamine drugs can inhibit this effect (Crunkhorn and Willis, 1971). Nanogram doses of PGE_1 or PGE_2 also cause pronounced erythema when injected intradermally in rabbit, rat, or man (for review, see Willis et al., 1972).

In view of this evidence, it was decided to investigate whether the release of prostaglandins from platelets would explain the nature of a platelet permeability factor (Smith and Willis, 1970). The action of thrombin on washed platelets was selected for the initial study because that action had been examined in great detail (for review, see Holmsen, Day, and Stormorken, 1969). Suspensions of washed human platelets were incubated for five minutes with thrombin or saline and extracts subsequently made. Prostaglandin-like activity in the extracts was quantitated by use of the rat fundus-strip and rat colon superfused in cascade with Krebs solution containing a mixture of antagonists to block the effects of acetylcholine, serotonin, histamine, and the catecholamines. Challenged with extracts of thrombin solution or saline-treated platelet suspension, neither of these tissues gave any indication of the presence of prostaglandins. But challenged with extracts of platelet preciably. Prostaglandin-like activity had therefore been developed by platelets in response to thrombin. To estimate how much of this activity was released from platelets, supernatant and pellet fractions of thrombin-treated platelet suspension incubated with thrombin, both contracted ap-suspensions were prepared and extracts made. Extracts of the supernatant fraction contracted the rat fundus and rat colon, and the responses were similar to those caused by extracts of the whole-platelet suspension. On the other hand, extracts of the pellet fraction had little effect. Most of the prostaglandin-like activity developed by platelets was therefore *released* from them. Thin-layer chromatography of extracts of thrombin-treated platelet suspension indicated that the prostaglandin-like material was largely PGE_2, although some $PGF_{2\alpha}$ was also present.

The results of the initial study have been confirmed by studies supported by radioimmunoassay (Silver, Smith, *et al.*, 1972; Smith, Silver, *et al.*, 1972). These studies carried out with platelet-rich plasma, show that (like thrombin) collagen, adrenaline, and ADP induce prostaglandin formation. The relative abilities of these various agents to induce prostaglandin formation in platelet-rich plasma is illustrated in Figure I-1. The finding that PGE_2 can be both synthesized by and released from platelets lends strong support, when coupled with its potent inflammatory action, to the hypothesis that this prostaglandin is a platelet permeability factor.

Protein

Nachman, Weksler, and Ferris (1970) discovered that isolated human-platelet granules (presumably lysosomes) con-

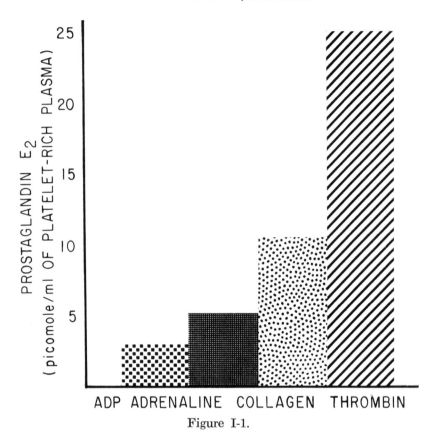

ADP ADRENALINE COLLAGEN THROMBIN

Figure I-1.

tain a heat-stable, cationic protein which increases vascular permeability. The protein is similar to the cationic protein found in leukocytes by Seegers and Janoff (1966). Some permeability effects of this platelet protein are inhibited by antihistamines, and the protein itself is mastocytolytic. Neither whether the protein is released from platelets during degranulation nor whether it contracts the guinea-pig ileum was determined.

Further research on the nature of this protein (Nachman, Weksler, and Ferris, 1972) revealed that it had a molecular weight of about 30,000 and produced a biphasic increase in vascular permeability in rabbit skin. The acute (15-minute) increase in vascular permeability was blocked by anti-histamines, but the delayed (three-hour) permeability effect was not, indeed, being characterized by leukocyte infiltration. It is possible that the cationic platelet protein is phospholipase A, an enzyme known to liberate histamine from mast cells (Uvnäs, 1963); this would explain the acute effect of the platelet protein. Furthermore, phospholipase A is known to trigger the synthesis of prostaglandins by liberating their fatty-acid precursors from cell-membrane phospholipid. The delayed effect of the platelet protein would then be explained by the production of endogenous PGE_2. It has been suggested that phospholipase A from the lysosomes of leukocytes plays an important role in carrageenan-induced inflammation (Anderson, Brocklehurst, and Willis, 1971), and a relatively heat-stable phospholipase A with an optimum acid pH and a molecular weight of 55,000 has been identified in brain tissue (Cooper and Webster, 1972). Platelets contain and release a similar enzyme (Smith, Silver and Webster, 1973).

PROSTAGLANDINS AND ASPIRIN

Willis (1969) demonstrated that PGE_2 is present in inflammatory exudate induced by carrageenan in the rat and suggested that it is a mediator of that reaction. The appearance of prostaglandin in exudate is delayed for about two and a half hours after carrageenan injection. There is then an infiltration of polymorphonuclear leukocytes, together with an associated swelling; both are inhibited by nonsteroidal anti-inflammatory drugs (Di Rosa and Willoughby, 1971). If this delayed response is mediated by PGE_2, aspirin-like drugs could act by suppressing its accumulation. Since aspirin inhibits the release of permeability factors from platelets, it was decided to examine the effects of anti-inflammatory drugs on the thrombin-induced formation and release of prostaglandins from platelets (Smith and Willis, 1971). In experiments *in vitro*, drugs were added to suspensions of washed human platelets two minutes before the addition of thrombin. Prostaglandins were then extracted and bioassayed. Aspirin, in concentrations as low as $1\mu g/ml$, reduced the production of prostaglandins by platelets. This finding would seem to be of great importance in view of the potency of aspirin. Indomethacin was even more effective than aspirin, but sodium salicylate was much less effective, and hydrocortisone was without effect.

Using homogenates of guinea-pig lung, Vane (1971) independently demonstrated that the conversion of arachidonic acid into prostaglandins is inhibited by indomethacin, aspirin, or sodium salicylate. The potency ratings, on a weight basis, were 368, 16, and 1, respectively. Inhibition of prostaglandin synthesis by indomethacin or aspirin has also been demonstrated in isolated perfused dog spleen (Ferreira, Moncada, and Vane, 1971) and preparations of sheep seminal vesicles (Smith and Lands, 1971; Tomlinson *et al.*, 1972). In view of these findings, it is almost certain that one action of aspirin-like drugs on platelets is inhibition of prostaglandin synthetase.

Smith and Dawkins (1971) have pointed out that the "demonstration that salicylate, or indeed any drug, inhibits the activity of an enzyme *in vitro* is not sufficient evidence that one or more of the *in vivo* actions of the drug are due to such inhibition." In an attempt to obviate such a criticism of the effect of aspirin on prostaglandin production, *in vivo* studies were undertaken (Smith and Willis, 1971). Blood was taken immediately before and one hour after subjects ingested two tablets (600 mg) of aspirin; suspensions of washed platelets from both bleedings were then simultaneously incubated with thrombin. The supernatants from the thrombin-treated platelet suspensions were extracted for prostaglandins and the extracts bioassayed as described previously. Extracts from the "before-aspirin" suspensions showed prostaglandin activity equivalent to that of about 100 pmole of PGE_2, whereas extracts from the "after-aspirin" suspensions showed prostaglandin activity equivalent to that of less than 10 pmole of PGE_2. Consequently, the release of prostaglandins from platelets in response to thrombin had been inhibited by 90 percent or more by the oral administration of therapeutic doses of aspirin. When the subjects received no drugs or only codeine (100 mg), release of prostaglandins was found to be unaltered; but, when the subjects received indomethacin (50 or 100 mg), release of pro-staglandins was considerably reduced. The action of aspirin was very specific. Aspirin had no effect on the thrombin-in-duced release of serotonin, adenine nucleotides, or lysosomal enzymes, which are recognized constituents of platelet granules. It may be concluded that an *in vivo* action of aspirin-like drugs is inhibition of prostaglandin biosynthesis.

These findings reinforce the proposition that PGE_2 is a platelet permeability factor and provide a rationale for the use of aspirin in inflammatory conditions in which prostaglandins have been identified, such as contact dermatitis (Greaves, Søndergaard, and McDonald-Gibson, 1971), inflammation of the eye (Ambache, 1961), and burn syndrome (Anggard and Jonsson, 1972). Possible implications of inhibition of pro-staglandin synthesis by aspirin-like drugs have been discussed in detail by Vane (1971) and by Collier (1971), although neither author mentions hemostasis. It has been known for several years that aspirin prolongs normal bleeding time and can lead to serious bleeding when a patient has a coagulation dis-order. It is possible that this action of aspirin is related to inhibition of the production of prostaglandins by plate-lets.

SUMMARY

The evidence detailed above supports the speculation that platelets participate in some inflammatory reactions. Platelets can release permeability factors, including pro-staglandin E_2, in response to thrombin, collagen, or ADP. They have also been shown to contain a cationic protein which increases permeability. The direct active Arthus reaction has an absolute requirement for platelets (Mar-garetten, 1972), and the way in which they may partic-ipate in this reaction has been discussed by McKay (1972). Thrombophlebitis, an inflammatory condition in which veins are occluded by a thrombus, may involve the re-lease of platelet prostaglandins (Silver, Smith, *et al.*, 1972).

Therapeutic doses of aspirin suppress the production of prostaglandin E_2 by platelets. Aspirin also inhibits the prosta-glandin synthetase of several tissues. These observations support the view that prostaglandin E_2 mediates the various inflammatory reactions in which its presence has been demonstrated and give rise to the speculation that prostaglandins play some part in hemostasis.

REFERENCES

Ambache, N.: Prolonged erythema produced by chromatographically purified irin. *J Physiol (Lond), 160:* 3, 1961.

Anderson, A. J., Brocklehurst, W. E., and Willis, A. L.: Evidence for the role of lysosomes in the formation of prostaglandins during carrageenan-induced inflammation in the rat. *Pharm Res Commun, 3:* 13, 1971.

Anggard, E., and Jonsson, C. E.: Efflux of prostaglandins in lymph from scalded tissue. *Acta Physiol Scand, 81:* 440, 1971.

Bergström, S., Carlson, L. A., and Weeks, J. R.: The prostaglandins: a family of biologically active lipids. *Pharmacol Rev, 20:* 1, 1968.

Collier, H. O. J.: Prostaglandins and aspirin. *Nature, 232:* 17, 1971.

Cooper, M. F., and Webster, G. R.: On the phospholipase-A_2 activity of human cerebral cortex. *J Neurochem, 19:* 333, 1972.

Cotran, R. A.: The delayed and prolonged vascular-leakage inflammation. II. An electron microscopic study of the vascular response after thermal injury. *Am J Pathol, 46:* 589, 1965.

Crunkhorn, P., and Willis, A. L.: Cutaneous reactions to intradermal prostaglandins. *Br J Pharmacol, 41:* 49, 1971.

David-Ferreira, J. F.: The blood platelet: electron-microscopic studies. *Int Rev Cytol, 17:* 99, 1964.

Day, H. J., Holmsen, H., and Hovig, T.: Subcellular particles of human platelets. *Scand J Haematol (Suppl), 7:* 1, 1969.

Di Rosa, M., and Willoughby, D. A.: Screens for anti-inflammatory drugs. *J Pharm Pharmacol, 23:* 297, 1971.

Ferreira, S. H., Moncada, S., and Vane, J. R.: Indomethacin and aspirin abolish prostaglandin release from the spleen. *Nature [New Biol], 231:* 237, 1971.

Greaves, M. W., Søndergaard, J., and McDonald-Gibson, W.: Recovery of prostaglandins in human cutaneous inflammation. *Br Med J, 2:* 258, 1971.

Holmsen, H., Day, H. J., and Stormorken, H.: The blood-platelet-release reaction. *Scand J Haematol (Suppl), 8:* 1, 1969.

Hovig, T.: The ultrastructure of blood platelets in normal and abnormal states. *Ser Haematol, I, 2:* 3, 1968.

Humphrey, J. H., and Jaques, R.: The histamine and 5-hydroxytryptamine content of platelets and leukocytes in various species. *J Physiol* (Lond.), *124:* 305, 1954.

Marcus, A. J., and Zucker, M. B.: *The physiology of blood platelets.* New York, Grune, 1965.

Margaretten, W.: Quoted in McKay, D. G.: Participation of components of the blood-coagulation system in the inflammatory response. *Am J Pathol, 67:* 181, 1972.

McKay, D. G.: Participation of components of the blood-coagulation system in the inflammatory response. *Am J Pathol, 67:* 181, 1972.

Mustard, J. F., and Packham, M. A.: Platelet phagocytosis. *Ser Haematol, I, 2:* 168, 1968.

Mustard, J. F., Movat, H. Z., MacMorine, D. R. L., and Senyi, A.: Release of permeability factors from the blood platelet. *Proc Soc Exp Biol Med, 119:* 988, 1965.

Nachman, R. L., Weksler, B., and Ferris, B.: Characterization of human-platelet vascular-permeability-enhancing activity. *J Clin Invest, 51:* 549, 1972.

Nachman, R. L., Weksler, B., and Ferris, B.: Increased vascular permeability produced by human-platelet-granule cationic extract. *J Clin Invest, 49:* 274, 1970.

Packham, M. A., Nishizawa, E. E., and Mustard, J. F.: Response of platelets to tissue injury. *Biochem Pharmacol (Suppl),* page 171. London, Pergamon, 1968.

Pletscher, A.: Metabolism, transfer, and storage of 5-hydroxytryptamine in blood platelets. *Br J Pharmacol Chemother, 32:* 1, 1968.

Seegers, W., and Janoff, A.: Mediators of inflammation in leukocyte lysosomes. VI. Partial purification and characterization of a mast-cell-rupturing component. *J Exp Med, 124:* 833, 1966.

Silver, M. J., Smith, J. B., Ingerman, C., and Kocsis, J. J.: Blood prostaglandins: Formation during clotting. *Prostaglandins, 1:* 428, 1972.

Smith, J. B., and Willis, A. L.: Formation and release of prostaglandins by platelets in response to thrombin. *Br J Pharmacol, 40:* 545, 1970.

Smith, J. B., and Willis, A. L.: Aspirin selectively inhibits prostaglandin production in human platelets. *Nature [New Biol], 231:* 235, 1971.

Smith, J. B., Silver, M. J., Ingerman, C., and Kocsis, J. J.: Prostaglandin production during platelet aggregation. *III Congress, International Society on Thrombosis and Haemostasis, 1972.*

Smith, J. B., Silver, M. J., and Webster, G. R.: Phospholipase A_1 of human blood platelets. *Biochem. J. 131:* 615, 1973.

Smith, M. J. H., and Dawkins, P. D.: Salicylate and enzymes. *J Pharm Pharmacol, 23:* 729, 1971.

Smith, W. L., and Lands, W. E. M.: Stimulation and blockade of prostaglandin biosynthesis. *J Biol Chem, 246:* 6700, 1971.

Tocantins, L. M.: The mammalian blood platelet in health and disease. *Medicine (Baltimore)*, *17*: 155, 1938.

Tomlinson, R. V., Ringold, H. J., Qureshi, M. C., and Forcheilli, E.: Relationship between inhibition of prostaglandin synthesis and drug efficacy: Support for the current theory on mode of action of aspirin-like drugs. *Biochem Biophys Res Commun*, *46*: 552, 1972.

Uvnäs, B.: Mechanism of histamine release in mast cells. *Ann NY Acad Sci*, *103*: 278, 1963.

Vane, J. R.: Inhibition of prostaglandin synthesis as a mechanism of action for aspirin-like drugs. *Nature [New Biol]*, *231*: 232, 1971.

Willis, A. L.: Release of histamine, kinin, and prostaglandins during carrageenan-induced inflammation in the rat. In Mantegazza, P., and Horton, E. W. (Eds.): *Prostaglandins, Peptides and Amines.* London, Acad Pr, 1969.

Willis, A. L., Davison, P., Ramwell, P. W., Brocklehurst, W. E., and Smith, J. B.: Release and actions of prostaglandins in inflammation and fever: inhibition by anti-inflammatory and antipyretic drugs. In Ramwell, P. W., and Pharriss, B. B. (Eds.): *Prostaglandins in Cellular Biology,* Alza Conference Series. New York, Plenum Pr, 1972, Vol. 1.

CHAPTER II

WHITE BLOOD CELLS AND CRYSTAL-INDUCED INFLAMMATION*

H. Ralph Schumacher

THE ACUTE SYNOVITIS of both gout and pseudogout is characterized by synovial effusion loaded with polymorphonuclear leucocytes (PMN). In experimental monosodium-urate-crystal-induced arthritis in the dog, PMN are also prominent and have been shown to be essential for full expression of the joint inflammation (Phelps and McCarty, 1966).

Electron micrographs (EM) of synovial-fluid PMN in human gout show evidence of degranulation, necrosis of some cells, and loss of phagosomal membranes (Fig. II-1). Schemes to explain the pathogenesis of acute gouty arthritis (McCarty, 1965) have suggested that crystals released from deposits in avascular tissue are phagocytized by PMN, which may perpetuate the inflammation by release of lactic acid, lysosomal enzymes, or both. It has also been suggested that crystal-laden PMN die and release their crystals to be phagocytized again.

In order to examine the sequence of crystal-PMN reaction *in vitro*, the author and his associates have studied human PMN incubated with synthetic urate crystals from three minutes to two hours (Schumacher and Phelps, 1971). The crys-

* This work was supported in part by research funds from the Veterans Administration, Barsumian Memorial Fund, NIH grant AN-12593 and FR-107, VA TR-39, and grant RR-40 from the General Clinical Research Resources, NIH.

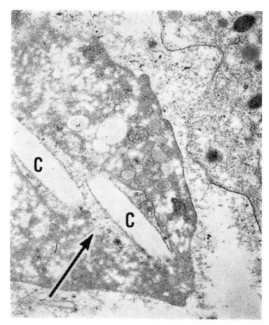

Figure II-1. Electron micrograph of synovial-fluid PMN from patient with acute gouty arthritis. C = crystals in phagosomes. Portions of the phagosomal membrane are lost (arrow). There is diffuse loss in cytoplasmic density. (25,000 ×.)

tals are phagocytized (Fig. II-2) and, at first, lie within the phagosomes, very close to the phagosomal membranes. Some dense bodies empty into the phagosomes (Fig. II-3). In other areas, phagolysosome lysis seems to occur without definite evidence of dense-body fusion with the phagosome. Degranulation increases with time. Twenty percent of the PMN are necrotic (as defined by EM) within thirty minutes (Fig. II-4); 50 percent are dead at the end of two hours. Thus urate crystals can have a profound and rapidly toxic effect on isolated human PMN. The rapid release of crystals and enzymes from necrotic cells certainly can tend to perpetuate the inflammation. A chemotactic factor is also released by PMN during a period about the same as that just mentioned (Phelps, 1970).

The mechanisms for the toxic effect of monosodium-urate crystals on PMN are not yet established. The closeness of

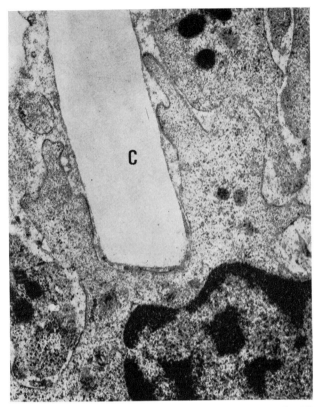

Figure II-2. PMN-cell processes enfolding urate crystal (C) at the beginning of phagocytosis. (28,000 ×.)

the crystals to the phagosomal membrane raises the possibility that the crystals may injure the membrane. Wallingford and McCarty (1971) have shown that monosodium-urate crystals can lyse erythrocyte membranes *in vitro*. Sodium urate, like silica, which breaks down macrophage phagosomes (Allison, Harrington, and Birbeck, 1966) is a hydrogen donor.

Electron micrographs also suggest other possible mechanisms, including later phagosome distention and lysosomal-enzyme reaction with the crystals. An osmotic effect during the distention could also damage the phagosome. Phagosomal-membrane lysis does seem to be part of the sequence leading to cell death, but the exact sequence has not yet been defined.

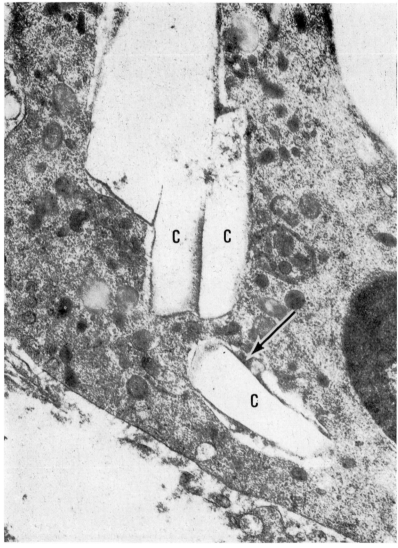

Figure II-3. Urate crystals (c) in PMN after thirty minutes of incubation *in vitro*. Portions of the crystal lie very close to the phagosomal membrane, which is not well defined at some parts. Note the dense material (arrow), probably from dense bodies (lysosomes) lying adjacent to one crystal. (32,000 ×.)

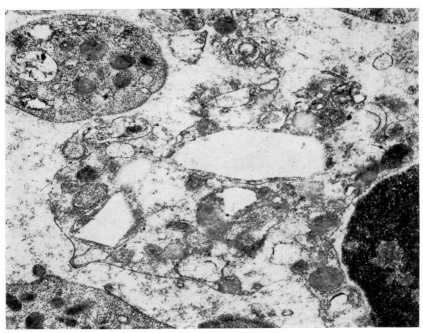

Figure II-4. Necrotic PMN thirty minutes after mixing of urate crystals and human leucocytes. The cell membrane is no longer definable, and cytoplasmic components are released into the surrounding medium. (32,000 ×.)

Although some bacteria may lyse phagosomal membranes (Armstrong and Sward, 1966), most bacteria, immune complexes, and other particles do not seem to (Weissman, *et al.,* 1971).

Urate crystals do not have the same rapid toxic effect on mononuclear phagocytes.

After making the above-mentioned studies with urates, the author and his associates examined, *in vitro,* calcium-pyrophosphate-crystal phagocytosis in the same system. The crystals were prepared by Dr. Rose Tse as described elsewhere (Tse and Phelps, 1970). These crystals are said not to be hydrogen donors (Weissman, 1971). Under polarized light, they proved slightly larger than but otherwise similar to human crystals.

X-ray diffraction showed almost pure calcium-pyrophosphate dihydrate, although electron microscopy revealed what seemed to be some contamination with hydroxyapatite-like crystals. Despite larger doses of crystals, there was a lesser degree of phagocytosis (Schumacher and Phelps, unpublished). After two hours, 22 percent of the PMN contained crystals, as compared to 50 percent in the experiments with the urates. Only 8 percent of the cells were dead. Of the cells with identifiable crystals, 23 percent proved necrotic in the calcium-pyrophosphate studies, as compared to 71 percent in the urate

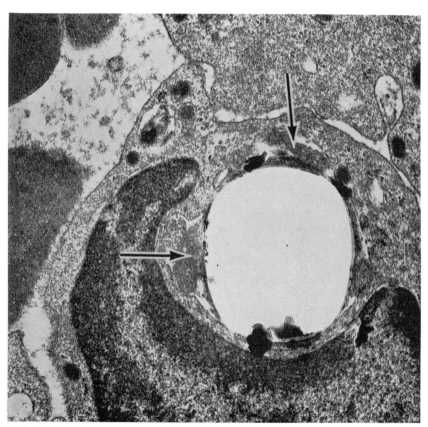

Figure II-5. After two hours incubation, dense calcium-pyrophosphate crystals although fragmented in the cutting, are still in an intact phagosome of a viable PMN. The arrows show material from dense bodies lying with the crystal (c) in the phagosome. (29,000 ×.)

studies. Although the pyrophosphate crystals were often dislodged and produced some artefacts, the phagosomal membranes were otherwise largely intact (Fig. II-5). Dense bodies emptied into the phagosomes, but the degree of degranulation was much less than in the parallel studies with urates. Some phagosomes were very much dilated, as in human pseudogout (Bluhm, *et al.*, 1969), but some crystals were also very close to the phagosomal membranes. This different handling of pyrophosphate crystals by PMN is supported by studies (Wallingford and Trend, 1971) showing that urate but not calcium-pyrophosphate crystals produce lysis of erythrocyte membranes. Release of cytoplasmic as well as lysosomal enzymes occurs after

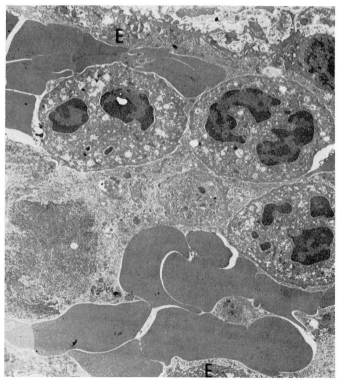

Figure II-6. Degranulation of intraluminal PMN. This example is from a patient with acute arthritis of unknown etiology. PMN have few dense bodies and many lucent areas in the cytoplasm. E = endothelium. (5,000 ×.)

in vitro phagocytosis of urate crystals but not of calcium-pyrophosphate crystals (Andrews and Phelps, 1971. Whether the slight difference in crystal size is important in the different handling has not been examined.

In *vivo*, these crystals are also apparently handled differently (McCarty, 1970). Synovial-exudate cells in gout often show no distinct phagosome membranes around the urate crystals, whereas, in pseudogout, easily demonstrable phagosomes occur. Whether calcium pyrophosphate, unlike urate, is not a hydrogen donor and whether that is the reason for the different handling remains to be determined.

In gout, PMN need not phagocytize crystals in order to degranulate. In fact, in both human gout and experimental urate-crystal synovitis in dog knees, degranulation of PMN in synovial-vessel lumens has been observed (Schumacher and Agudelo, 1972) (Fig. II-6). The full role of such intraluminal degranulation has yet to be explored. Both urate and pyrophosphate crystals are also phagocytized by synovial-lining cells (Agudelo and Schumacher, 1971; Agudelo, Schumacher, and Phelps, 1972; and Schumacher, 1968). Sequential studies of urate-crystal synovitis (Agudelo, Schumacher, and Phelps, 1972) in the dog model suggest that this is an earlier finding and may even contribute the first chemotactic factor that attracts PMN to the joint (Fig. II-7).

In dog joints injected with sodium-urate crystals, joint motion clearly accentuates the intensity of inflammation (Agudelo, Phelps, and Schumacher, 1972). Whether this increases blood flow and brings more PMN to the joint, damaging PMN and releasing more enzymes; produces more crystal cell contact; changes temperature or pH; or acts in still other ways is under study.

Because the anti-inflammatory effect of colchicine in gout (but probably not in pseudogout) is said to work, at least in part, by dissolving microtubules (Malawista and Bensch, 1967), the author and his associates have examined, using the same *in vitro* system described earlier (Schumacher and Phelps, 1971), urate-crystal-and-leucocyte interaction with and without incubation of the leucocytes with colchicine 10^{-8}M or indo-

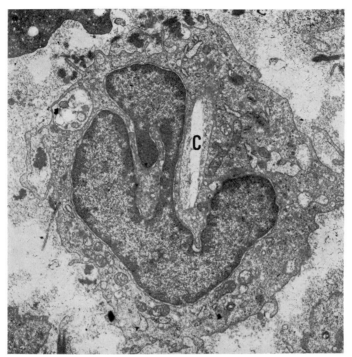

Figure II-7A. Urate crystal (c) in phagosome of probable synovial-lining cell from the synovial fluid. (10,000 ×.)

methacin 10^{-6}M. The studies made showed microtubules infrequently demonstrable in PMN, although easily demonstrable in lymphocytes and monocytes. Colchicine had no effect on number of microtubules or microfilaments; amount of cytoplasmic degranulation or material from dense bodies in phagosomes; number of pseudopods; number of cells with crystals or number of crystals per cell; morphology of the phagosome; or number of necrotic cells.

The synovial-fluid cells of one patient with acute gouty arthritis were examined before the patient had received any treatment and one, two, and twenty-four hours after he received 3 mg of intravenous colchicine that produced excellent symptomatic relief of his condition. No detectable change in the cells or their handling of the crystals (Fig. II-8) could be found. Interestingly, neither before nor after the patient received

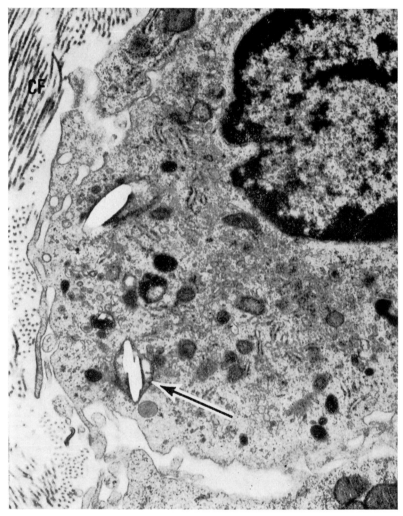

Figure II-7B. Residual clefts from calcium-pyrophosphate crystals in phagosome (arrow) of lining cell in synovial membrane. CF = collagen. (15,000 ×.)

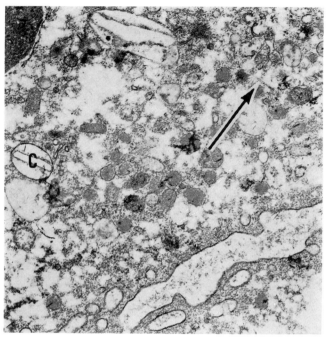

Figure II-8. One of the infrequent PMN microtubules (arrow) seen either before or after administration of 3 mg of intravenous colchicine to a patient with acute gout. This figure shows the microtubule one hour after administration of colchicine. C = crystals in phagosomes. (22,000 ×.)

the colchicine did his synovial-fluid PMN show more than 8 percent of the cells necrotic by EM (Fig. II-9). There were many examples of crystals apparently free in the cytoplasm of what seemed to be viable cells. In crystal-induced arthritis in the dog, the author and his associates have also seen few necrotic synovial-fluid PMN, despite crystal phagocytosis by 30 to 40 percent of the PMN at the end of four hours. The number of dead cells *in vivo* is thus far smaller than the number produced in the above-mentioned *in vitro* studies; and this raises several possibilities. The principal point is that varying amounts of crystals will obviously produce different effects. Current *in vitro* work with .4 mg of urate crystals/ml instead of 1 mg/ml is not producing the same profuse cell necrosis

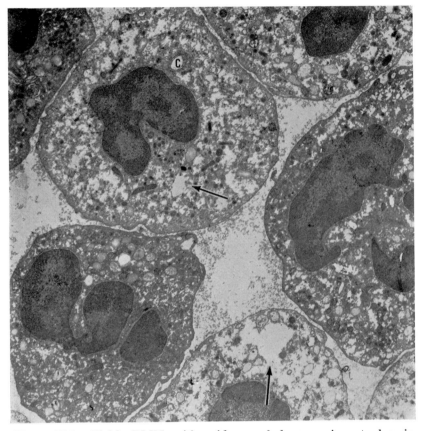

Figure II-9. Viable PMN, with evidence of decrease in cytoplasmic dense bodies in acute gouty synovial fluid, as seen with or without presence of colchicine. Some urate crystals (c) lie in phagosomes, but other sites (arrows) suggest that phagosomal membranes may have broken down. (22,000 ×.)

(Andrews and Phelps, 1971; Andrews and Schumacher, work in progress). The number of crystals released into a joint in acute gout may thus determine whether lysosomal-enzyme release from viable cells or necrosis of cells is predominant. Certainly, some necrotic cells *in vivo* are phagocytized by monocytes and lining cells (Fig. II-10); and this may make the counts of necrotic cells not exactly comparable with those made in the *in vitro* situation. The *in vitro* studies referred

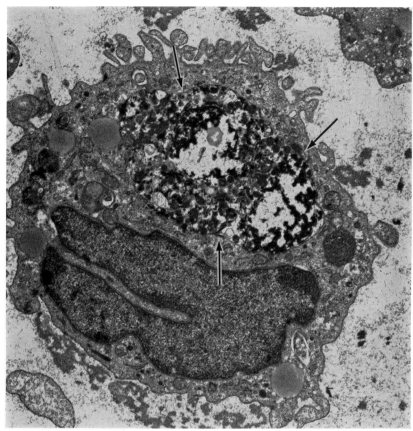

Figure II-10. Synovial-exudate mononuclear cell containing phagocytized necrotic PMN (arrow) before administration of colchicine to patient. (16,000 ×.)

to have been done with normal PMN: conceivably, gouty PMN may handle crystals differently.

The absence of demonstrable effects on the PMN after clinically effective doses of colchicine in the patient and after *in vitro* doses of colchicine calculated to approximate clinically obtainable levels is felt to be important because of the emphasis of Wallace, Omokuku, and Ertel (1970) on the point that the investigator must keep in mind in making *in vitro* studies, the drug levels that may be achieved *in vivo*. Negative ultrastructural studies cannot prove anything about the mode of action of colchicine but do serve to emphasize that its mechanism or mechanisms remain incompletely understood. Some effects of colchicine in varying doses on phagocytosis of certain particles, lysosomal-enzyme release, PMN motility, chemotaxis, formation of digestive vacuoles, PMN adherence, and the kallikrein system have been shown in different systems (Malawista and Andriole, 1968).

Colchicine *in vitro* at $10^{-8}M$ or in clinically effective intravenous doses produced no detectable changes in PMN that were phagocytizing urate crystals. This suggests that the action of colchicine may be on the mechanisms that attract or exude the PMN into the joint rather than on the crystal-cell reaction in the joint space.

SUMMARY

Polymorphonuclear leucocytes are necessary for the full-blown acute arthritis of gout and probably for full expression of pseudogout. The PMN handle the two synthetic crystals quite differently, dramatic PMN necrosis being produced by urates but not by even larger doses of calcium pyrophosphate.

Whether this difference is due to the hydrogen-donor status of the crystal or to some other property is not yet clear. The urate-crystal effect on PMN appears to be dose-dependent.

The PMN may also contribute to the inflammation by undergoing intraluminal degranulation before making contact with the crystal. Other cells, such as synovial-lining cells, may also be important in initiating the inflammation.

Since colchicine produces no detectable morphologic changes in PMN when they phagocytize urate crystals, it may exert much of its effect on the mechanism exuding PMN into the joint.

REFERENCES

Agudelo, C., and Schumacher, H. R.: The synovial membrane in acute gouty arthritis: a light- and electron-microscopic study. *Arthritis Rheum, 14:* 147–148, 1971.
Agudelo, C., Phelps, P., and Schumacher, H. R.: Effect of exercise

on urate-crystal-induced inflammation in canine joints. *Arthritis Rheum, 15:* 100, 1972.

Agudelo, C., Schumacher, H. R., and Phelps, P.: Sequence of synovial changes in urate-crystal-induced arthritis in the dog. *Arthritis Rheum, 15:* 108–109, 1972.

Allison, A. C., Harrington, J. S., and Birbeck, M.: An examination of cytotoxic effects of silica on macrophages. *J Exp Med, 124:* 141–154, 1966.

Andrews, R., and Phelps, P.: Release of lysosomal enzymes from polymorphonuclear leucocytes following phagocytosis of monosodium-urate and calcium-pyrophosphate-dihydrate crystals: effect of colchicine and indomethacin. *Arthritis Rheum, 14:* 368, 1971.

Andrews, R., and Schumacher, H. R.: Study of nitrobluetetrazolium in crystal phagocytosis. Work in progress.

Armstrong, B. A., and Sward, C. P.: Electron microscopy of listeria-monocytogenes-infected mouse spleen. *J Bacteriol, 91:* 1346–1355, 1966.

Bluhm, G. B., Riddle, J. M., Barnhart, M. I., Duncan, H., and Sigler, J. W.: Crystal dynamics in gout and pseudogout. *Med Times, 97:* 135, 1969.

Malawista, S. E., and Andriole, V. T.: Colchicine: anti-inflammatory effect of low doses in a sensitive bacterial system. *J Lab Clin Med, 72:* 933–942, 1968.

Malawista, S. E., and Bensch, K. G.: Human polymorphonuclear leucocytes: demonstration of microtubules and effect of colchicine. *Science, 156:* 521–522, 1967.

McCarty, D. J.: Crystal-induced inflammation of the joints. *Ann Rev Med, 21:* 357, 1970.

McCarty, D. J.: The inflammatory reaction to microcrystalline sodium urate. *Arthritis Rheum, 8:* 726–735, 1965.

Phelps, P.: Polymorphonuclear leucocytes motility *in vitro.* IV. Colchicine inhibition of chemotactic-activity formation after phagocytosis of urate crystals. *Arthritis Rheum, 13:* 1–9, 1970.

Phelps, P., and McCarty, D. J.: Crystal-induced inflammation in canine joints. II. Importance of polymorphonuclear leucocytes. *J Exp Med, 124:* 115–126, 1966.

Schumacher, H. R.: The synovitis of pseudogout: electron-microscopic observations. *Arthritis Rheum, 11:* 426–435, 1968.

Schumacher, H. R., and Agudelo, C.: Intravascular degranulation of neutrophils: an important factor in inflammation? *Science, 175:* 1139–1140, 1972.

Schumacher, H. R., and Phelps, P.: Sequential changes in human polymorphonuclear leucocytes after urate-crystal phagocytosis: an electron-microscopic study. *Arthritis Rheum, 14:* 513–526, 1971.

Tse, R. L., and Phelps, P.: Polymorphonuclear leucocyte motility *in vitro*. V. Release of chemotactic activity following phagocytosis of calcium-pyrophosphate crystals, diamond dust, and urate crystals. *J Lab Clin Med, 76:* 403–415, 1970.

Wallace, S. L., Omokuku, B., and Ertel, N. H.: Colchicine-plasma levels: implications as to pharmacology and mechanism of action. *Am J Med, 48:* 443–445, 1970.

Wallingford, W. R., and McCarty, D. J.: Differential membranolytic effects of microcrystalline sodium urate and calcium pyrophosphate dihydrate. *J Exp Med, 133:* 100–112, 1971.

Wallingford, W. R., and Trend, B.: Phagolysosome rupture after monosodium-urate but not calcium-pyrophosphate-dihydrate phagocytosis *in vitro*. *Arthritis Rheum, 14:* 420, 1971.

Weissman, G.: The molecular basis of acute gout. *Hosp Pract, 6:* 43–52, 1971.

Weissman, G., Zurier, R. B., Spieler, P. J., and Goldstein, I.: Mechanisms of lysosomal-enzyme release from leucocytes exposed to immune complexes and other particles. *J Exp Med, 134:* 1495–1655, 1971.

CHAPTER III

THE ROLE OF SERUM COMPLEMENT

IN NEUTROPHIL-MEDIATED

INFLAMMATION

MICHAEL E. NORMAN

HISTORICAL PERSPECTIVE

A DISCUSSION OF THE ROLES of serum complement and neutrophils in inflammation should begin with a brief historical review.

When Metchnikoff, in 1887, observed the attraction of leukocytes towards certain bacteria and their eventual ingestion, it had been known for some time that the presence of leukocytes was an important feature of the inflammatory response. The attraction of various chemical substances for leukocytes was clearly defined in the plant kingdom, and Leber, in 1888, using a capillary-tube technique in the cornea and anterior chamber of the rabbit eye, demonstrated a similar phenomenon in animals. It was Leber, too, who first used the term *chemotaxis* and stimulated intensive investigative efforts to define a whole host of chemotactic substances, among them whole bacteria and bacterial products, serum factors, and inflammatory products from injured tissues.

With the rapid advance of new knowledge of leukocyte function, a number of important questions were raised that continue to trouble investigators today:

1. Does the presence of leukocytes (specifically, neutrophils) in inflammatory sites represent active, directional migration

of cells, random cellular movement, or inhibition of cellular movement?

2. Are there specific chemotactic factors for different cell types and would this explain the observation of sequential or particular cell appearances in different inflammatory lesions?

3. What are the mechanisms governing cellular migration?

Early investigators recognized the difficulty of correlating histologic examinations with the nature of a leukocyte response *in vivo*. In 1936, using bacterial stimuli and a dark-ground photographic-tracer technique, McCutcheon and his colleagues showed directional migration of neutrophils. On the other hand, aseptically induced injury in the rabbit-ear chamber gave rise to an accumulation of leukocytes that could not be correlated with directional migration. Unexplained but clearly important was the role of vascular-permeability mediators in initiating cell movement.

This brings us to a consideration of the role of the complement system. Metchnikoff believed that the leukocyte played the dominant role in a final common pathway of host defense—namely, phagocytosis of an offending antigen. At the turn of the century, however, Wright and Douglas (1903) defined the role of certain humoral factors, labelled "opsonins," which did not seem to be antibodies but were essential for enhancement of particle uptake. As initially defined, opsonins were heat-labile, serum-derived materials; it is now well established that this was an oversimplification, for current data include multiple classes of heat-labile and heat-stable opsonins that are both species- and particle-specific.

A gap in understanding the inflammatory response was closed when serum was demonstrated to play a role in physically joining antigens, antibodies, and inflammatory cells. Sequential analysis revealed that the first four complement components mediated this reaction of immune adherence, C3 playing the dominant role. And it was only after the isolation and purification of individual components that, using sensitized sheep red-blood cells, Gigli and Nelson (1968) demonstrated the requirement of these same components in a phagocytic system. About the same time, Johnston and his coworkers (1969) confirmed complement mediation in the *in vitro* phagocytosis of pneumococcal organisms.

THE COMPLEMENT SYSTEM

Table III-I shows the nine basic components of the complement system. C1 consists of three subunits, requiring complex interaction for activation. Not shown are the naturally occurring inhibitors of C1, C3, and C6. These proteins fall into the *beta*-globulin class, with the exception of $C1_q$, which is a gammaglobulin. Stepwise activation of the complement sequence displays immunochemical and kinetic behavior characteristic of enzyme-substrate interactions. The immunochemical characterization and separation of the complement components has been a fruitful but exceedingly complex process. In the analysis of structure-function relationships, investigators have turned to the biologic functions of the system (Fig. III-I):

Three basic pathways of function are illustrated:

1. The traditional or classic "cascade" sequence shows stepwise activation of all nine components, resulting in injury to cell membranes and eventual cell death. This reaction pattern is the basis of the procedure for titrating hemolytic complement, the amount of which reflects the integrity of the entire system. It should be noted that complement functions in other biologic assays, and quantitative measurements of individual components, do not correlate well with hemolytic titres in many experimental and clinical settings. Indeed, Bladen and his colleagues (1967) have proved that comple-

TABLE III-I
PROPERTIES OF COMPLEMENT COMPONENTS

Component	Serum concentration (ug/ml)	Approx. Mol. Wt.
C1q	190	400,000
r	—	—
s	22	79,000
C2	20–40	117,000
C3	1,200	185,000
C4	430	240,000
C5	75	200,000
C6	15	—
C7	15	—
C8	10	150,000
C9	10	79,000

PATHWAYS OF COMPLEMENT ACTIVATION

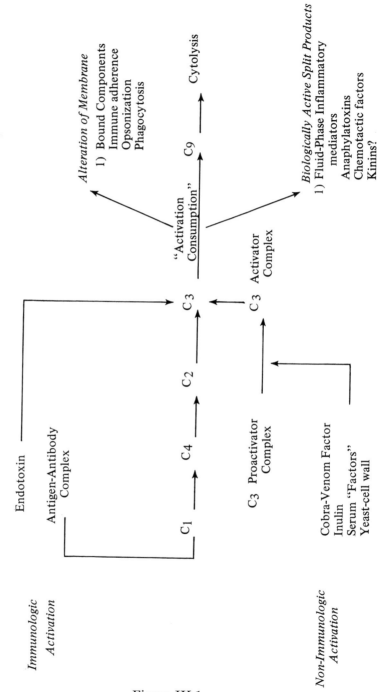

Figure III-1.

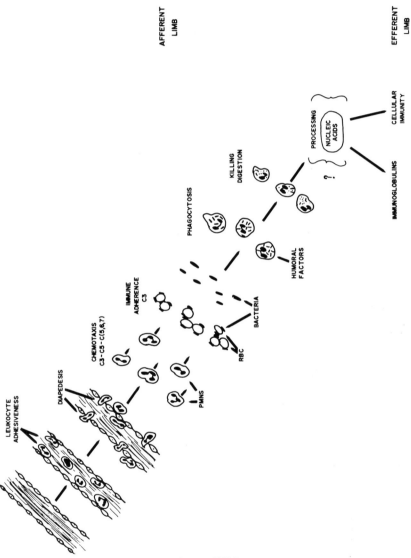

Figure III-2.

ment activation may proceed by alternative pathways, bypassing the first three components, when purified endotoxin is added to fresh serum in certain biologic assays. The relationship of this observation to clinical endotoxemia is under vigorous investigation at present. Using purified cobra-venom factor and other materials, Müller-Eberhard (1967) has shown a similar activation sequence.

2. Complement activation and layering of components on the cell membrane, in bound form, alters its biologic characteristics and may or may not result in eventual cytolysis. Immune adherence and phagocytosis are representative examples of this phenomenon.

3. During the sequence of complement activation, fragments of native components are split off; these have potent biologic activity. Of particular importance are the chemotactic factors, which will be discussed further.

Figure III-2 shows the multiple roles of complement in the inflammatory response. This sequence of reactions is called the "afferent limb" of immune function.

IMMUNOLOGIC REACTIONS AND INFLAMMATION

The production of inflammation by immunologic reactions and their by-products is well known (Table III-II).

TABLE III-II
RELATIONS OF INFLAMMATION AND IMMUNOLOGIC REACTIONS*

I. Production of inflammation by immunologic reactions and immunologically active substances
  A. Initiated by antigen-antibody interaction
  B. Produced by 1) preformed antigen-antibody complexes
              2) immunoglobulins and products thereof
              3) the complement system and products thereof
II. Enhancement or production of immunologic reactions by and during inflammation
  A. Generation or release of auto-antigens
  B. Stimulation of immunologically active cells
  C. Activation of the complement system
III. Development of chronic from acute inflammation: caused by
  A. Retained antigen
  B. Auto-antigen

* Published by permission of Dr. Michael Reynolds.

The complement system functions through at least four general mechanisms in producing inflammation (Table III-III).

TABLE III-III
RELATIONS OF INFLAMMATION AND IMMUNOLOGIC
REACTIONS*

Refer to I, B, 3, in Table III-II: Produced by the complement system and products thereof
1. Chemotactic activity
2. Release of a) mast-cell amines
         b) serum-chemotactic factors
3. Promotion of phagocytosis
4. Immune adherence

* Published by permission of Dr. Michael Reynolds.

The understanding of how inflammation and immunologic reactivity interrelate through complement requires a discussion of what has recently been learned about neutrophil-complement cooperation.

LEUKOCYTE-COMPLEMENT INTERACTIONS

The development of experimental animal models to assess the interaction of leukocytes and serum complement in the inflammatory response was stimulated by the vital work of Stephen Boyden. In 1962, he described a method of assessing the separate cellular and humoral contributions to neutrophil chemotaxis *in vitro*. Boyden observed that the migration of rabbit neutrophils through a millipore filter required the presence of heat-labile factor(s) in fresh guinea-pig serum. Since that time, many modifications of the Boyden chamber have been devised, such as the one illustrated in Figure III-3 and in current use in our laboratory. Migration of cells is an energy-dependent process requiring membrane deformability as the cells squeeze through the filter towards a chemotactic stimulus. After ap-

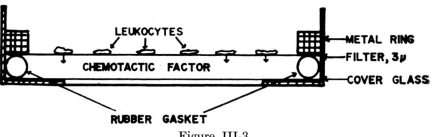

Figure III-3.

propriate incubation, fixing, staining, and mounting of the filter, the number of cells on the attractant side are counted. Results may be expressed as a ratio or as the average number of cells per high-power field.

Despite Boyden's suggestion that complement was involved in the phenomenon, Keller and Sorkin (1965) challenged its role, demonstrating chemotaxis at pH gradients inhibitory of complement function. Between 1965 and 1968, data derived from inflammation models in rat, rabbit, and guinea pig firmly established the link between complement and chemotactically active materials in serum (Unanue and Dixon, 1967; Cochrane, 1968).

Arthus Phenomenon

Ward and Cochrane (1965) inhibited the development of local hemorrhagic vasculitis (e.g., Arthus reaction) in rabbits by complement inactivation or removal, and by the induction of neutropenia, without effects on other neutrophil-mediated functions. The role of complement-bound immune complexes deposited in local vessels was supported by histologic and immunofluorescent studies. As mentioned previously, the interpretive significance of these findings depended on recognizing species-specificity and cross-reactivity of complement components.

Nephrotoxic Glomerulonephritis

Cochrane and his associates correlated proteinuria, glomerular-tuft neutrophil counts, and complement binding with glomerular basement membrane (GBM) in acute nephrotoxic glomerulonephritis (Fig. III-4). Notice that, in Figure III-4, a complement-independent, alternative pathway of injury is indicated, without participation of complement or neutrophils, at least in the acute phase. The concept of a biphasic pattern in this form of acute inflammation is characterized by a secondary or "autologous" phase of immunologic reactivity. Production of host antibody to heterologous proteins occurs after the acute inflammatory response, as glomerular neutrophil counts fall and serum complement rises towards

COMPLEMENT-MEDIATED NEUTROPHIL INJURY
IN NEPHROTOXIC GLOMERULONEPHRITIS

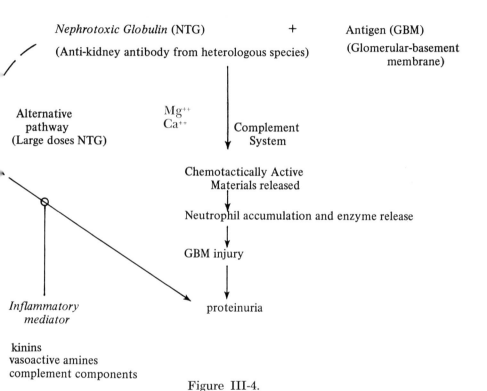

Figure III-4.

normal values. Some years ago, a scheme of the events leading to organ-specific injury was postulated by Dr. Frank Dixon (1967) in his model of the nephritis in which antibodies attack the basement membrane of the glomerulus (Fig. III-5). With the exception of the nephritis in Goodpasture's syndrome, however, the significance of this model in clinical disease has not been proved.

Serum Sickness and Immune-Complex Nephritis

The production of soluble immune complexes upon intravenous administration of antigen leads to the arteritis of serum

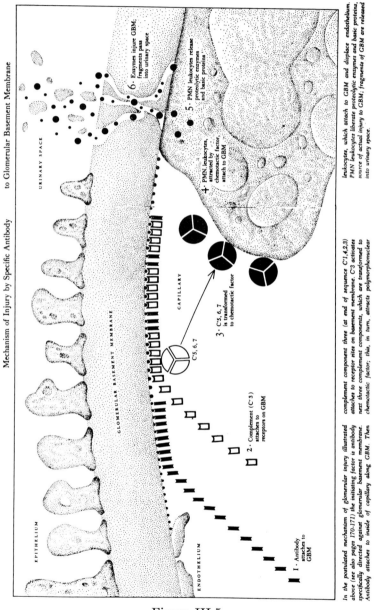

Figure III-5.

In the postulated mechanism of glomerular injury illustrated above (see also pages 170-171) the initiating factor is antibody specifically directed against glomerular basement membrane. Antibody attaches to inside of capillary along GBM. Then complement component three (at end of sequence C'1,4,3) attaches to receptor sites on basement membrane. C'3 activates next three complement components, which are transformed to chemotactic factor; this, in turn, attracts polymorphonuclear leukocytes, which attach to GBM and displace endothelium. PMN leukocytes liberate proteolytic enzymes and basic proteins, source of actual injury to GBM; fragments of GBM are released into urinary space.

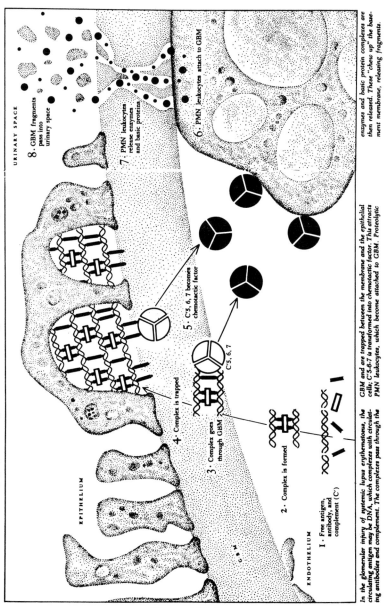

Figure III-6.

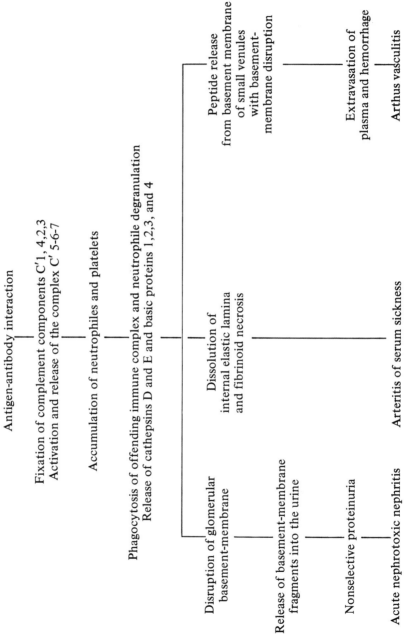

Figure III-7. Mediators associated with development of acute immunologic injury in experimental animal models.

sickness and immune-complex nephritis. Figure III-6 shows the deposition of immune complexes along the glomerular basement membrane, followed by complement binding and activation, chemotactic-factor generation, and subsequent accumulation of neutrophils with release of cell constituents and basement-membrane injury.

Localization and deposition of complexes seem to require a combination of altered hemodynamic forces and release of vasoactive substances from platelets and injured tissues (Kniker and Cochrane, 1968). An unanswered question is how chemotactic gradients, essential for one-way directional migration, are established in free-flowing vessels. Also unexplained is the selective inhibition, by neutrophil depletion, of necrotizing arteritis, but not glomerulonephritis, in acute serum sickness in the rabbit model. A summary of these models is shown schematically in Figure III-7. The clinical significance of immune-complex nephritis is more firmly grounded; examples include acute post-streptococcal glomerulonephritis, lupus-erythematosus nephritis, and the nephritides associated with syphilis and malaria.

What are the chemotactically active complement components? Current data from a number of laboratories point to biologically active split fragments of the third and fifth components ($C3_a$ and $C5_a$, respectively) and a large trimolecular complex C567 (Keller and Sorkin, 1965; Snyderman *et al.*, 1968, 1969, 1970; Taylor and Ward 1967; Ward, Cochrane and Müller-Eberhard, 1965, 1966; Ward, 1967). The multiplicity of techniques employed in chemotactic-factor generation is illustrated in the next three tables (Tables III-IV, III-V, III-VI). I emphasize this point because it highlights the impressive heterogeneity of pathway activation within the complement system.

Worthy of mention is work by Ward and Becker (1967) on intrinsic mechanisms of neutrophil movement. Activation of serine esterases on or in the neutrophil surface was found, with C567 as the chemotactic stimulus, to be a requirement for cell migration and could be inhibited by phosphonate esters.

TABLE III-IV
COMPLEMENT FACTORS POSSIBLY INVOLVED
IN CHEMOTAXIS OF NEUTROPHILS IN VITRO*

Factor	Approx. mol. wt.	Method of formation	Comments and references
C3 split product	6,000	Streptokinase + plasminogen (− plasmin) + C3 Streptokinase + plasminogen (− plasmin) + serum	Chemotactic but not anaphylactic; Ward (76)
		Streptokinase + plasminogen (− plasmin) + serum	No evidence for chemotactic activity; Stecher and Sorkin (72)
C3 split product	—	Purified C3 + trypsin	Weak chemotactic activity; Ward and Newmann (83)
C3 split product	14,000	Purified C3 + tissue protease Serum + tissue protease	Hill and Ward (25)
C3a	7,000–8,700	Purified C3 + trypsin Purified C3 + C3 convertase Purified C3 + C3 inactivator complex Purified C3 + plasmin	Chemotactic and anaphylatoxic act.; Bokisch et al. (3)
C3a	10,000	Whole guinea-pig serum + LPS Purified C3 + EAC 142	Not chemotactic but anaphylatoxic activity; Shin et al. (67)
C3a	10,000	Fresh serum + Ag/Ab Fresh serum + LPS	Primarily anaphylatoxic activity; Mayer et al. (46)

* From Sorkin, E. J., Stecher, V. J. and Borel, J. F.: Chemotaxis of leukocytes. *Ser Haematol*, 3: 142 (Table II), 1970. Reprinted with permission of publisher.

TABLE III-V*
COMPLEMENT FACTORS POSSIBLY INVOLVED IN CHEMOTAXIS OF NEUTROPHILS IN VITRO*

Factor	Approx. mol. wt.	Method of formation	Comments and references
C5	15,000	Purified C5 + EAC 1423	Chemotactic and anaphylatoxic; Shin et al. (65)
C5 split product	8,500	Purified C5 + trypsin Purified C5 + EAC 1423	Chemotactic but not anaphylatoxic; Ward and Newmann (83)
C5 split product	15,000	Purified C5 + trypsin	Chemotactic and anaphylatoxic; Jensen et al. (30)
C5 split product	15,000	Guinea-pig serum + cobra-venom factor	Chemotactic and anaphylatoxic; Shin et al. (66)
C5a	15,000	Guinea-pig serum + LPS	Chemotactic and anaphylatoxic; chemotactic activity decreased by rabbit anti-C5 but not anti-C3; Snyderman et al. (69)
C5a	15,000	Fresh serum + LPS Fresh serum + Ag/Ab	Chemotactic and anaphylatoxic; Mayer et al. (46)

* From Sorkin, E. J., Stecher, V. J. and Borel, J. F.: Chemotaxis of leukocytes. *Ser Haematol, 3*: 142 (Table II), 1970. Reprinted with permission of publisher.

TABLE III-VI*
COMPLEMENT FACTORS POSSIBLY INVOLVED IN CHEMOTAXIS OF NEUTROPHILS IN VITRO*

Factor	Approx. mol. wt.	Method of formation	Comments and references
C(567)	200,000	Interaction of purified C components C1-7	C5, 6 and 7 necessary for chemotactic activity; Ward et al. (81)
		C6 deficient rabbit serum + Ag/Ab C6 deficient rabbit serum + LPS Anti-C6 serum from C6-deficient rabbit + Ag/Ab Anti-C6 serum from C6-deficient rabbit + LPS	C6-deficient sera react identical to NRS in chemotaxis experiments. Anti-C6 has no effect on activity; thus presence of C6 in serum not important for activation by Ag/Ab or LPS; Stecher and Sorkin (72)
		Anti-C6 rabbit antibody + normal rabbit serum + Ab/Ab	Depression of chemotactic activity from 100%–40%, depending on serum; Ward (77a)
		Whole rabbit or human or guinea-pig serum + Ag/Ab or endotoxin	Chemotactic factor is low mol. wt. product: Snyderman et al. (69). C5a accounts for most of PMN chemotactic activity; Mayer et al. (46)
Relation to C not defined	5,000–35,000	Normal rabbit serum	Chemotactic for neutrophils; Keller and Sorkin (37), Wilkinson et al. (84)

* From Sorkin, E. J., Stecher, V. J. and Borel, J. F.: Chemotaxis of leukocytes. *Ser Haematol, 3*: 142 (Table II), 1970. Reprinted with permission of publisher.

Borel, Keller and Sorkin (1969) and Hurley (1964) have characterized cellular responses in immunologic inflammation requiring the release of subcellular chemotactically active materials at the time of phagocytosis.

MECHANISMS OF NEUTROPHIL INJURY

Henson's studies (1971) focus on release of neutrophil contituents as the mechanism of injury. The process can be viewed graphically, as in Table III-VII. Table III-VII shows 1) two separate pathways binding neutrophils to immune complexes (it is important to note that both the complement- and immunoglobulin-mediated pathways seem to function whether or not phagocytosis takes place) and 2) degranulation and release occurring in a similar but alternative fashion.

TABLE III-VII

MECHANISMS OF RELEASE OF NEUTROPHIL (PMN)
CONSTITUENTS IN TISSUE INJURY

STEP I: PMN's + Immune Complexes

A) *Complement-mediated*
    1) Complement fixation to particles or surfaces (RBC, Zymosan, filter)
    2) Immune adherence of PMN's, with or without subsequent phagocytosis
        a) Inhibition by trypsin, chelation, complement removal
        b) C3 as component of central importance, with or without subsequent phagocytosis

B) *Immunoglobulin-mediated*
    1) Immunoglobulin fixation to particles or surfaces
    2) Immune adherence of PMN's with or without subsequent phagocytosis: enhanced in presence of large, insoluble, aggregated immunoglobulin precipitates
            IgG_{1-4} + IgM —
            IgA + IgD —

STEP II: Degranulation and Release of Constituents

           "two-step process"
A. Phagocytosis————————————→ enzyme release
    1) Release of enzymes into phagocytic vacuole
    2) Opening of vacuole to outside of cell

B. Binding to nonphagocytosable membrane (micropore filter) ——→ enzyme release
    1) Direct degranulation of cell to the outside; no lysis
    2) Sequential release demonstrated (?)

C. Enzyme release: active process requiring
    1) PMN energy-producing metabolism
    2) Serine esterases
    3) Calcium
    4) Cyclic-AMP (?)

BIOLOGIC SIGNIFICANCE FOR MAN

Evidence for complement participation in human disease is based on three observations:

1. depression of hemolytic-complement titres in serum, or quantitative measurements of individual components
2. *in vivo* fixation of bound complement in diseased tissues
3. increased catabolism of complement components

The interpretation of complement disturbances in immunologic inflammatory disease is subject to certain qualifications. The presence of bound or fluid-phase components in local inflammatory sites may not be reflected in serum alterations, and the converse is sometimes true. The relative insensitivity of serum complement, particularly to localized processes of consumption, is illustrated in the active rheumatoid joint, or in the cerebrospinal fluid in lupus erythematosus of the central nervous system. Complement levels are usually normal in serum but are markedly reduced in the synovial and spinal fluids.

Few studies have evaluated synthetic and metabolic rates of individual complement components, but the need for metabolic-turnover studies of injected and radiolabelled purified components is clear. Alper and his colleagues (1970) in Boston have recently described a young man with recurrent infections, multiple abnormalities of *in vitro* complement-mediated functions, and a markedly increased catabolic rate of injected C3. In certain forms of immunologically mediated glomerulonephritis, preliminary studies suggest, decreased complement synthesis offers an alternative explanation for the depressed serum-complement levels, which, according to the traditional view, result from activation and deposition of a complex (antigen, antibody, and complement) within the glomerulus.

In recent years, several genetically determined, biosynthetic defects of complement have been described. These include:

1. defects in naturally occurring inhibitors, resulting in spontaneous consumption of components
2. congenital absence of a complement component or components
3. synthesis of a functionally defective component

Hereditary angioneurotic edema is an autosomal-dominant disorder in which the serum lacks inhibitory factor against C1 esterase, a condition due either to absence of inhibitor protein or to presence of an inactive analogue (Donaldson and Evans, 1963).

Congenital absence of the second and third complement components has been described in man (Alper *et al.*, 1968; Cooper, TenBensel and Kohler, 1968; Klemperer *et al.*, 1966; and Klemperer, Austin and Rosen, 1967). Discovery of the absence of the fifth component in inbred strains of mice by Rosenberg and Tachibana (1962) and Nilsson and Müller-Eberhard (1965) and of the sixth component in rabbits has provided a valuable tool in complement research (Rother *et al.*, 1966).

It is striking that, as first described, absence of these components should occur without clinical disease. This observation has prompted further analysis of the relationship between quantitative levels and functional capacity of individual components.

Miller and his coworkers, in 1968 and 1970, using an *in vitro* assay of yeast-particle phagocytosis, have made the critical observation that a functional abnormality of the fifth component is associated, in man, with devastating clinical disease. This syndrome is shown in Table III-VIII. Of particular significance is the rather narrow spectrum of offending organisms. Vital to our understanding of structure-function relationships are Drs. Miller and Nilsson's findings of normal quantitative levels of C5 in the patients studied and of normal results in other biologic assays of complement in the

TABLE III-VIII
SYNDROME OF DEFICIENCY OF FIFTH
*COMPONENT OF COMPLEMENT**

1. Inflammatory dermatitis (seborrheic, eczema-like)
2. Failure to thrive almost from birth
3. Diarrhea
4. Severe recurrent bacterial infections, especially of gram-negative type
5. Normal peripheral WBC counts and intracellular killing
6. Normal cellular and humoral immunity
7. Opsonic deficiency of plasma, resulting in markedly reduced phagocytosis
8. Mixed inheritance patterns (autosomal dominant or recessive)
9. Marked response to fresh plasma infusions

* Published by permission of Dr. Michael E. Miller.

patients' serum. In addition, the clinical entity discovered confirms previous data showing different opsonic requirements for different antigens. What remains to be established is the convincing separation of humoral contributions by other biologic functions to phagocytosis in a given *in vitro* assay.

The question of specific neutrophil defects in inflammatory disease has generated vigorous investigative work in the last decade. The cellular contributions to complement-mediated inflammatory responses may be regulated by activation of specific receptors on the neutrophil. It is possible that discrete and separable neutrophil functions, such as chemotaxis and random mobility, are receptor-dependent for initiation. At present, a controversy exists over the validity of measurements of random mobility as a distinct and more primitive form of leukocyte movement. So far, the clinical significance of this function is unproved.

In both clinical and experimental settings, however, Miller and Nilsson (1971) have demonstrated specific cellular-movement defects that may occur independently. A number of metabolic inhibitors that suppress chemotaxis do not, for example, affect random mobility. The relationship between neutropenia, disorders of neutrophil chemotaxis and mobility, and "nature's experiments" are illustrated in Table III-IX. The lazy-leukocyte syndrome is characterized by defective chemotaxis and random mobility in the face of normal complement function (Miller, Oski and Harris, 1971). Furthermore, when comparisons are made with normal neutrophil mobility in other forms of neutropenia, its significance becomes more convincing. Another group of patients, currently under study,

TABLE III-IX
LAZY-LEUKOCYTE SYNDROME*
1) Recurrent stomatitis, gingivitis, otitis media, and fever
2) Normal humoral and cellular immunity
3) Severe neutropenia, usually less than 400 PMN's/mm³
4) Normal morphologic picture and numbers of mature PMN's in marrow
5) Poor PMN response to epinephrine and Piromen (e.g., "marginal pool")
6) Poor inflammation on Rebuck skin window
7) Normal PMN phagocytosis (yeast particles) and killing
8) Poor marrow and inadequate chemotaxis of peripheral blood
9) Poor random mobility of PMN's

* Published by permission of Dr. Michael E. Miller.

display congenital ichthyosis, chronic T.-rubrum infection, and selective deficiency of chemotaxis. These disorders seem to be inherited. Finally, Miller (1971) has shown that neutrophils from healthy newborns demonstrate a consistent and highly significant deficiency in response to a multiplicity of chemotactic factors. This is probably a defect of developmental immaturity and may explain, in part, the newborn's enhanced susceptibility to infection.

SUMMARY

We must recognize that complete understanding of the interaction of complement and neutrophils in inflammatory disease awaits sequential analysis of the entire inflammatory sequence in man.

REFERENCES

Alper, C. A., Abramson, N., Johnston, R. B., Jr., Jandl, J. H., and Rosen, F. S.: Increased susceptibility to infection associated with abnormalities of complement-mediated functions and of the third component of complement (C3). *N Engl J Med, 282:* 349, 1970.

Alper, C. A., Propp, R. P., Johnston, R. B., and Rosen, F. S.: Genetic aspects of human C′3 (abstract). *J Immunol, 101:* 816, 1968.

Bladen, H. A., Gewurz, H., and Mergenhagen, S. E.: Interactions of the complement system with the surface and endotoxic lipopolysaccharide of veillonella alcalescens. *J Exp Med, 125:* 767, 1967.

Borel, J. F., Keller, H. U., and Sorkin, E.: Studies on chemotaxis. XI. Effect on neutrophils of lysosomal and other subcellular fractions from leukocytes. *Int Arch Allergy, 35:* 194, 1969.

Boyden, S.: The chemotactic effect of mixtures of antibody and antigen on polymorphonuclear leukocytes. *J Exp Med, 115:* 453, 1962.

Cochrane, C. G.: Immunologic tissue injury mediated by neutrophilic leukocytes. *Advances Immun., 9:* 97, 1968.

Cochrane, C. G., Unanue, E. R., and Dixon, F. J., Jr.: A role of polymorphonuclear leukocytes and complement in nephrotoxic nephritis. *J Exp Med, 122:* 99, 1965.

Cooper, N. R., TenBensel, R., and Kohler, P. F.: Studies of an additional kindred with hereditary deficiency of the second component of human complement (C2) and description of a new method for the quantitation of C2. *J Immunol, 101:* 1176, 1968.

Dixon, F. J.: Glomerulonephritis and immunopathology. *Hospital Prac, 2:* 35, 1967.

Donaldson, V. A., and Evans, R. R.: A biochemical abnormality in hereditary angioneurotic edema—absence of serum inhibitor of C'1 esterase. *Am J Med, 35:* 37, 1963.

Gigli, I., and Nelson, R. A.: Complement dependent immune phagocytosis. I. Requirements for C'1, C'4, C'2, C'3. *Exp Cell Res, 51:* 45, 1968.

Henson, P. M.: Interaction of cells with immune complexes: adherence, release of constituents, and tissue injury. *J Exp Med, 134s:* 114, 1971.

Hurley, J. V.: Substances promoting leukocyte emigration. *Ann NY Acad Sci, 116:* 918, 1964.

Johnston, R. B., Jr., Klemperer, M. R., Alper, C. A., and Rosen, F. S.: The enhancement of bacterial phagocytosis by serum—the role of complement components and their cofactors. *J Exp Med, 129:* 1275, 1969.

Keller, H. U., and Sorkin, E.: Studies on chemotaxis. I. On the chemotactic and complement fixing activity of γ-globulins. *Immunology, 9:* 241, 1965.

Klemperer, M. R., Austen, F. K., and Rosen, F. S.: Hereditary deficiency of the second component of complement (C'2) in man: further observations on a second kindred. *J Immunol, 98:* 72, 1967.

Klemperer, M. R., Woodworth, H. C., Rosen, F. S., and Austen, K. F.: Hereditary deficiency of the second component of complement (C'2) in man. *J Clin Invest, 45:* 880, 1966.

Kniker, W. T., and Cochrane, C. G.: The localization of circulating immune complexes in experimental serum sickness—the role of vasoactive amines and hydrodynamic forces. *J Exp Med, 127:* 119, 1968.

Leber, T.: Über die Enstehung der Entzündung und die Wirkung der erregenden Schädlichkeiten. *Fortschr d Med, 6:* 460, 1888.

McCutcheon, M. and Dixon, H. M.: Chemotropic reactions of polymorphonuclear leukocytes to various microorganisms—a comparison. *Arch Pathol, 21:* 749, 1936.

Metchnikoff, E.: Sur la lutte des cellules de l'organisme contre l'invasion des microbes. *Ann Inst Pasteur, 1:* 321, 1887.

Miller, M. E.: Chemotactic function in the human neonate: humoral and cellular aspects. *Pediatr Res, 5:* 487, 1971.

Miller, M. E., and Nilsson, U. R.: A familial deficiency of the phagocytosis-enhancing activity of serum related to a dysfunction of the fifth component of complement. *N Engl J Med, 282:* 354, 1970.

———: Inhibition of chemotaxis by human leukocytes following incubation in homologous serum devoid of chemotactic activity (abstract). *J Immunol, 107:* 317, 1971.

Miller, M. E., Oski, F. A., and Harris, M. B.: Lazy-leukocyte syndrome—a new disorder of neutrophil function. *Lancet, 1:* 665, 1971.

Miller, M. E., Seals, J., Kaye, R., and Levitsky, L. C.: A familial, plasma-associated defect of phagocytosis. *Lancet, II:* 60, 1968.

Müller-Eberhard, H. J.: Mechanism of inactivation of the third component of human complement (C'3) by cobra venom. *Fed Proc, 26:* 744, 1967.

Nilsson, U. R., and Müller-Eberhard, H. J.: Isolation of β_{1F}-globulin from human serum and its characterization as the fifth component of complement. *J Exp Med, 122:* 277, 1965.

Rosenberg, L. T., and Tachibana, D.: Activity of mouse complement. *J Immunol, 89:* 861, 1962.

Rother, K., Rother, U., Müller-Eberhard, H. J., and Nilsson, U. R.: Deficiency of the sixth component of complement in rabbits with an inherited complement defect. *J Exp Med, 124:* 773, 1966.

Snyderman, R., Gewurz, H., and Mergenhagen, S. E.: Interactions of the complement system with endotoxic lipopolysaccharide—generation of a factor chemotactic for polymorphonuclear leukocytes. *J Exp Med, 128:* 259, 1968.

Snyderman, R., Phillips, J., and Mergenhagen, S. E.: Polymorphonuclear leukocyte chemotactic activity in rabbit serum and guinea pig serum treated with immune complexes: evidence for C5a as the major chemotactic factor. *Infect Immun, 1:* 521, 1970.

Snyderman, R., Shin, H. S., Phillips, J. K., Gewurz, H., and Mergenhagen, S. E.: A neutrophil chemotactic factor derived from C'5 upon interaction of guinea pig serum with endotoxin. *J Immunol, 103:* 413, 1969.

Taylor, F. B., and Ward, P. A.: Generation of chemotactic activity in rabbit serum by plasminogen-streptokinase mixtures. *J Exp Med, 126:* 149, 1967.

Unanue, E. R., and Dixon, F. J.: Experimental glomerulonephritis: immunological events and pathogenetic mechanisms. *Adv Immunol, 6:* 1, 1967.

Ward, P. A.: A plasmin-split fragment of C'3 as a new chemotactic factor. *J Exp Med, 126:* 189, 1967.

Ward, P. A., and Becker, E. L.: Mechanisms of the inhibition of chemotaxis by phosphonate esters. *J Exp Med, 125:* 1001, 1967.

Ward, P. A., and Cochrane, C. G.: Bound complement and immunologic injury of blood vessels. *J Exp Med, 121:* 215, 1965.

Ward, P. A., Cochrane, C. G., and Müller-Eberhard: Further studies on the chemotactic factor of complement and its formation *in vivo. Immunology, 11:* 141, 1966.

Ward, P. A., Cochrane, C. G., and Müller-Eberhard: The role of serum complement in chemotaxis of leukocytes *in vitro. J Exp Med, 122:* 327, 1965.

Wright, A. E., and Douglas, S. A.: An experimental investigation of the role of the blood fluids in connection with phagocytosis. *Proc R Soc Lond, 72:* 357, 1903.

CHAPTER IV

QUANTITATIVE STUDIES
OF INFLAMMATION
AND GRANULOMA FORMATION*

ROBERT S. SPEIRS and ELIZABETH E. SPEIRS

INTRODUCTION

THE INFLAMMATORY AREA and the regional lymph nodes make up the battleground upon which a motile population of blood leukocytes confronts bacteria and other foreign materials. The foreign material penetrates the body through a break in the epithelium and is generally prevented from spreading by an interlacing subepithelial mass of connective-tissue fibers. Within a short time, vasodilation occurs, and the area becomes perfused with fluid and cells from nearby blood vessels. The accumulated fluid, some foreign material, and pieces of cellular debris are channelled into lymphatic vessels and passed along to the regional lymph nodes, where filtration occurs. The cells taking part in these reactions are of a variety of types, each unique in its manner of development, its reaction to the foreign material, and its role in the resistance of the organism. Migration of these inflammatory cells to the inflamed area brings them into direct contact with the foreign material, or with other cells that have made contact with the material and are reacting to it. This is accompanied by a neu-

---

* This manuscript represents a review which includes the efforts of numerous coworkers who have contributed ideas and skills during the past 15 years. These include: Dr. Nicholas Ponzio, Dr. Thomas Athanassiades, Dr. Steven Paul, Dr. Matthew Turner, Mr. Jack Illari and Mr. Louis Lipsett.

tralization of toxic substances, phagocytosis, and eventual digestion or isolation of the material. In addition, a wide variety of cell-to-cell reactions takes place. Eventually, collagen formation occurs, as well as synthesis and secretion of immunoglobulins. Although many cells are consumed or destroyed in the local inflammatory reactions, others become activated and undergo morphological and functional changes. They leave the inflamed area and pass into the draining lymph nodes, eventually making their way back into the blood vessels by way of the thoracic duct. Concomitantly, cellular proliferation is induced locally as well as in the regional lymph nodes and in the central hemopoietic tissues.

Inflammation therefore initiates a new pattern of cellular traffic which is superimposed upon the normal circulation. It results in the loss of many preformed cells and the proliferation of new cells. The combined reactions of granulocytes, macrophages, lymphocytes, and associated cells culminate in states of tolerance, hypersensitivity, or immunity.

A knowledge of the different cells involved and an understanding of their reactions would permit a better understanding of the complex immunological states which evolve as a consequence of this exposure to antigen. This report describes ways in which these cells can be quantitatively studied *in vivo*. The eosinophil has been emphasized, since the manner of its reaction to antigen seems, in so many ways, unique.

QUANTITATIVE STUDIES OF THE INFLAMMATORY EXUDATE

Since inflammation involves a variety of different cells, each with its own rate of entry and exit, the types of cells present at the site vary at different times after inflammation has been induced. Sequential studies are therefore necessary to determine the overall reactions and understand the subsequent outcome. When inflammation is induced in solid tissue or within connective tissue, it is very difficult to do quantitative studies of the total cell population; and, in such cases, appraisals of the cellular reactions are usually based only on estimates of differential counts. Serious misinterpretations can arise.

This is illustrated in Figures IV-1 and IV-2, in which data from the same experiment to establish the effects of cortisone on blood neutrophils are plotted in two different ways. From Figure IV-1, it would seem that the tenfold increase in neutrophils (from 8 to 80) signified a substantial increase over the control levels. An entirely different impression results, however, from an examination of Figure IV-2. If the apparent increase is plotted as cells per cubic millimeter, it is obvious that the cortisone acetate had little effect on neutrophils *per se*. The percentage of change plotted in Figure IV-1 does not represent an actual increase in the number of neutrophils but is due to a decrease in the number of other cells.

When an inflammatory agent is introduced into the peritoneal cavity, the reacting cells are suspended in an induced exudate, and quantitative as well as qualitative techniques can be applied to estimate the total number of each type of cell present (Speirs and Dreisbach, 1956; Speirs, Speirs, and Jansen, 1961). The exudate is washed out with a known volume of diluent and quantitative estimates are made of the total cellular content. Differential counts may be made from smears of the exudate by routine blood-cell-staining procedures. The total number of each cell type is calculated as the product of the percentage and the estimated number of total cells.

The data shown in Figure IV-3 illustrate the sequential cellular reactions to an intraperitoneal injection of tetanus toxin. The left side shows the number of each type of inflammatory cell present when the antigen is neutralized and injected into nonimmunized mice. The right side charts the responses of animals previously immunized by subcutaneous injections of tetanus antigen.

In both groups, the neutrophils migrated very rapidly into the peritoneal cavity, becoming the predominant cells during the first day. They then decreased in number and were replaced by eosinophils and mononuclear cells. In nonimmunized mice, the eosinophils made up only a small component of the inflammatory exudate; but in immunized mice, relatively large numbers accumulated over a period from two to eight days. In both groups, the migration of mononu-

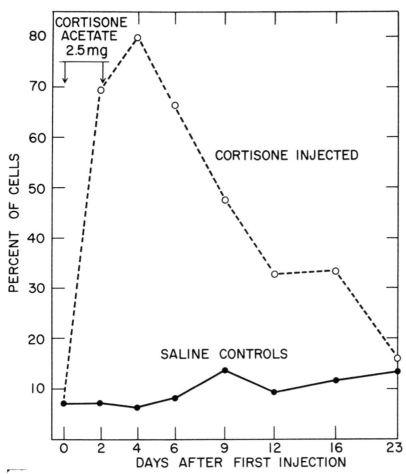

Figure IV-1. Leukocyte responses to subcutaneous injections of cortisone acetate. The percentage of neutrophils present in circulating blood after two subcutaneous injections of cortisone acetate in the mouse is shown. There was a ten-fold increase in the percentage of neutrophils, as against a much smaller increase of such cells in the saline-injected controls.

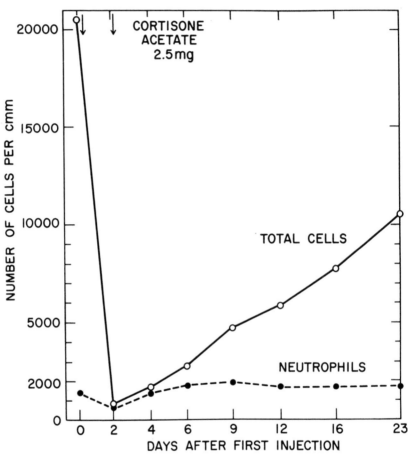

Figure IV-2. Leukocyte response to subcutaneous injections of cortisone acetate. Quantitative changes in the total number of leukocytes and neutrophils after two subcutaneous injections of cortisone acetate. The neutrophils decreased slightly in number on the second day but were otherwise unchanged. Although the data for plotting Figures IV-1 and IV-2 were taken from the same experiment, the interpretation of Figure IV-1 could be very misleading if quantitative counts had not been performed.

QUANTITATIVE RESPONSE

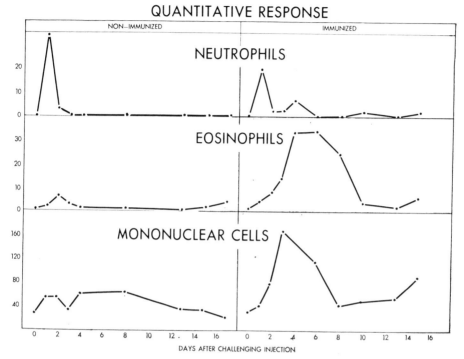

Figure IV-3. Estimate of number of cells in an inflammatory exudate induced by an intraperitoneal injection of tetanus toxin. The peritoneal cavity was flushed out with a known volume of diluent and routine hematological procedures applied. In the nonimmune animals (represented on the left), the toxin was first neutralized by antitoxin. Mice previously primed by subcutaneous injections of tetanus toxoid showed markedly higher eosinophil and mononuclear responses to challenge than did unprimed animals (Speirs, 1962).

clear cells began within twelve hours, and these cells eventually predominated in the exudate. A much greater mononuclear response was obtained in the immune animals. Marked morphological changes also occurred as these cells reacted to the specific antigen. Swelling, vesicle formation, blastoid changes, and an increase in cytoplasmic basophilia were observed.

Further studies were undertaken to correlate the number of eosinophils at the site of injection with the secondary rise in serum-antitoxin titres. The data shown in Figure IV-4

EOSINOPHIL RESPONSES AND SERUM ANTIBODY TITERS FOLLOWING A CHALLENGING INJECTION OF TETANUS TOXOID

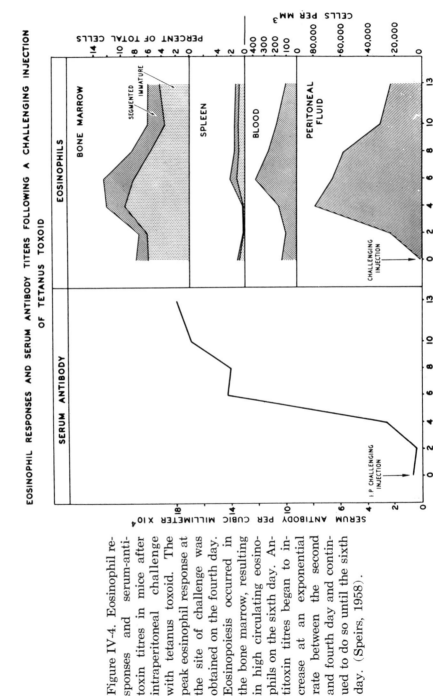

Figure IV-4. Eosinophil responses and serum-antitoxin titres in mice after intraperitoneal challenge with tetanus toxoid. The peak eosinophil response at the site of challenge was obtained on the fourth day. Eosinopoiesis occurred in the bone marrow, resulting in high circulating eosinophils on the sixth day. Antitoxin titres began to increase at an exponential rate between the second and fourth day and continued to do so until the sixth day. (Speirs, 1958).

EOSINOPHIL RESPONSES TO A RE - INJECTION OF TOXOID
(ABSOLUTE COUNTS)

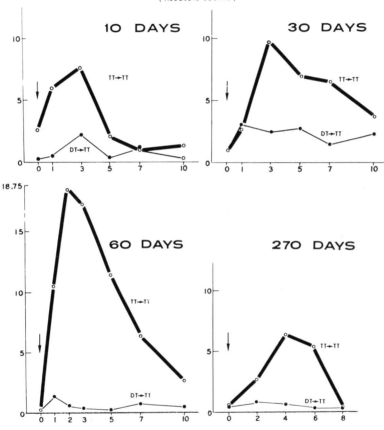

DAYS AFTER INJECTION

Figure IV-5. Eosinophil response to challenge at selected intervals after priming. The maximum eosinophil response was obtained with challenge sixty days after priming, but a significant response could still be obtained 270 days after priming. Control animals were primed with tetanus toxoid, but reinjected with diphtheria toxoid (Speirs and Speirs, 1964).

indicate that the increase in the eosinophils preceded by about two days the rise in antitoxin titres and that the number of eosinophils declined as the antitoxin titres peaked. In other areas examined (blood, bone marrow, and spleen) the eosinophils peaked on the sixth day when the number of eosinophils in the peritoneal fluid was declining.

Experiments using isotope-labelling procedures (tritiated thymidine) indicated that the precursors of eosinophils taking part in the inflammatory exudate had undergone DNA synthesis four to six days before the antigen challenge (Speirs, Jansen *et al.*, 1962). It is evident from the foregoing experiments that the intraperitoneal injection of antigen induced a marked shift of the population of mature eosinophils from the blood and spleen to the peritoneal cavity and that new eosinopoiesis was initiated to replace the cells lost. For a short period, there seemed to be an overcompensation of eosinophil proliferation, resulting in higher numbers of eosinophils in the bone marrow and in the circulation.

Figure IV-5 presents data obtained from animals primed to tetanus toxoid by subcutaneous injection, challenged intraperitoneally with either diphtheria or tetanus toxoid, and sacrificed at selected intervals. It may be noted that the capacity to mount an eosinophil response to the challenge persisted for long periods after the priming. The specificity of the response indicated that immunological memory must be involved; once formed, it presumably persists for the life of the animal.

Figure IV-6 illustrates that passive immunization did not increase the capacity to mount an eosinophil response to the challenge. In a series of experiments in which various combinations of isologous, homologous, and heterologous antitoxins were injected, no persistent local eosinophil response to the toxoid could be detected (Speirs and Wenck, 1955; Speirs, 1957).

On the other hand, as shown in Figure IV-7, a secondary type of eosinophil response was induced by adoptive transfer of lymph node or spleen cells from primed mice to normal or irradiated mice (Ponzio and Speirs, 1973; McGarry *et al.*, 1971). The experiments suggested that the accumulaiton of

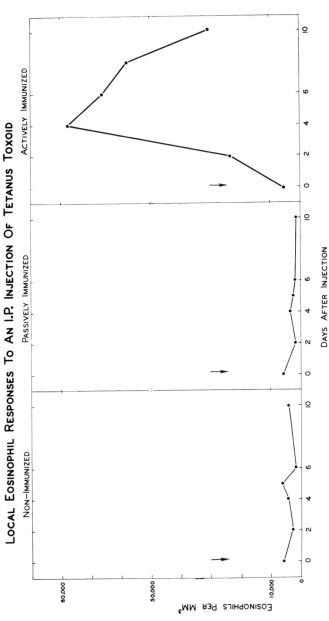

Figure IV-6. Eosinophil response to tetanus toxoid in nonimmunized, passively immunized and actively immunized mice. Passive transfer of immune serum did not give an eosinophil response (Speirs, 1958).

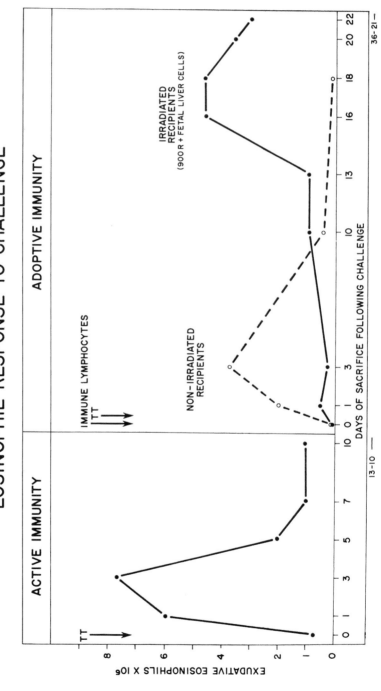

eosinophils is a manifestation of mediators released by specifically sensitized cells upon contact with the antigen.

To determine the effect of antitoxin on the eosinophil response, mice were primed subcutaneously by a single injection of tetanus toxoid and pertussis vaccine. This is known to induce sensitization without the formation of high antitoxin titres (Speirs and Turner, 1969). The animals were challenged intraperitoneally thirty days later. Before or after the challenging injection, they were injected intraperitoneally with isogeneic antitoxin and the eosinophil accumulations noted at selected intervals. Mice pretreated one or twenty-four hours before the challenge were inhibited in their capacity to mount an eosinophil response (Figure IV-8). On the other hand, when the antitoxin was administered twenty-four hours after the challenge, there was a secondary type of eosinophil response. There were no striking differences in the responses of either neutrophils or mononuclear cells.

These findings indicate that retention of eosinophils over a prolonged period—from three to seven days—is not dependent upon high levels of humoral antitoxin. Instead, high levels of antitoxin present at the time of challenge actually inhibit the eosinophil response.

In vitro studies of inflammatory cells demonstrated that eosinophils were chemotactically attracted to specific mononuclear cells (Speirs and Osada, 1962). The attraction resulted in the formation of cellular rosettes consisting of eosinophils around swollen vacuolated mononuclear cells (Figs. IV-9

←————————————————————————————————————

Figure IV-7. Eosinophil response following adoptive transfer of primed lymphoid cells. Spleen cells from mice primed to tetanus toxoid were injected into both normal and lethally irradiated reconstituted mice. A challenging injection of tetanus toxoid was given two hours later, and the animals were sacrificed at selected intervals. Nonirradiated animals showed an elevated eosinophil response between the first day and the third, returning to normal levels by the tenth day. Irradiated reconstituted mice were unable to respond for thirteen days, the time necessary for recovery of hemopoietic activity. At that time the newly formed eosinophils began to accumulate and large numbers remained at the site of antigen injection until after the 22nd day.

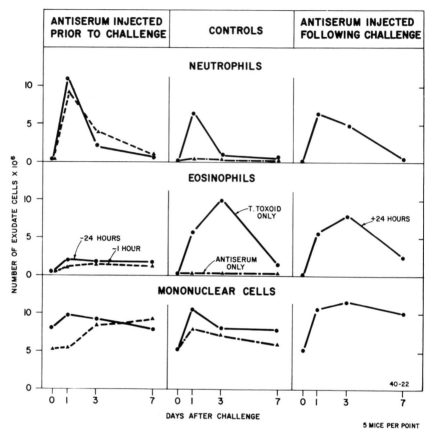

Figure IV-8. Effect of isologous tetanus antiserum on the cellular response to a challenging injection of tetanus toxoid. Intraperitoneal injection of antiserum either one or twenty-four hours before challenge markedly inhibited the eosinophil response but had no effect on neutrophils and only a slight effect on mononuclear cells. Antiserum given twenty-four hours after the challenging injection had no inhibitory effect upon the eosinophil response (Turner, Speirs, and McLaughlin, 1968).

and IV-10). These mononuclear cells contained antigen that seemed to trigger a release of mediators with a chemotactic effect for eosinophils (Speirs, 1962; Speirs and Speirs, 1963, 1964).

The inhibitory effect of humoral antibody on the eosinophil response described earlier would presumably be

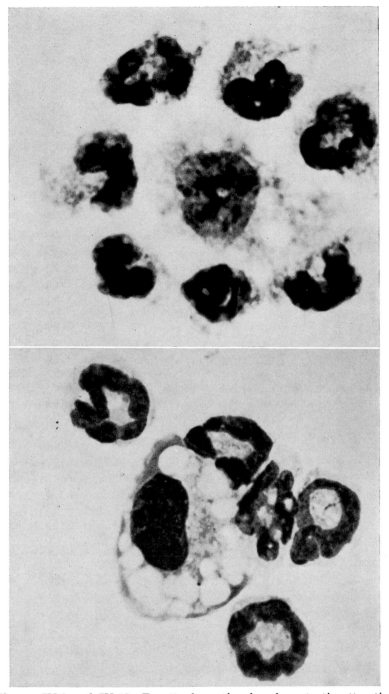

Figures IV-9 and IV-10. Rosette formation by chemotactic attraction
of eosinophils to mononuclear cells. Cells obtained from an inflammatory exudate induced by a challenging injection of tetanus toxoid were
cultured in Eagle's medium. Specific chemotactic attraction of eosinophils to swollen vacuolated mononuclear cells was observed.

due to its ability to complex with antigen before the antigen could activate the sensitized mononuclear cells to release eosinophilotactic substances.

STUDIES OF EXPERIMENTALLY INDUCED GRANULOMAS

It was noted that the inflammatory exudate induced in the peritoneal cavity by an injection of tetanus toxoid tended to subside after the first week. By the end of the second week, the number of cells present in the peritoneal cavity was similar to the number present in noninjected animals. At this time, serum antitoxin could first be detected and the titres continued to rise for the next six to eight weeks. This antitoxin was predominantly IgG, known to be secreted in large measure by plasma cells. Since plasma cells had not been observed in the inflammatory exudate, it was of interest to determine how and where they were formed.

Earlier, it had been observed that macrophages which engulfed antigenic material tended to clump together, often by intertwining their cytoplasmic processes (Fig. IV-11). Small aggregates of these cells, lymphoid cells, or both act as centers for the attachment of other inflammatory cells, forming cell masses which, by the third day, are visible to the naked eye (Fig. IV-12). These aggregates subsequently attach to the body wall or to the omentum, forming small nodules of granulomatous tissue. For the first week after induction of the inflammation, the cellular content of these aggregates is identical to that of the inflammatory exudate in the peritoneal cavity. Phagocytic cells are prominent; many contain lipid droplets; many become highly swollen and vacuolated or contain a disjointed rough endoplasmic reticulum with secretory material accumulated within the cisternae. These cells appear to undergo degeneration and necrosis.

As the inflammation within the peritoneal cavity subsides, the attached cellular aggregates persist and continue to show changes in cellular composition. By the seventh day, they are well organized with infiltration of blood-capillary sprouts which develop into arterioles, capillaries, and venules. Inflammatory cells continue to mi-

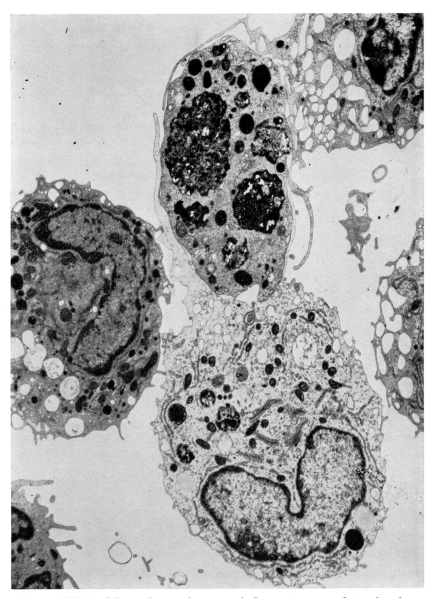

Figure IV-11. Macrophages from an inflammatory exudate showing formation of pseudopods which entwine themselves around cells containing phagocytized material. Small aggregates of such cells are observed during the first twenty-four hours after injection of the antigen.

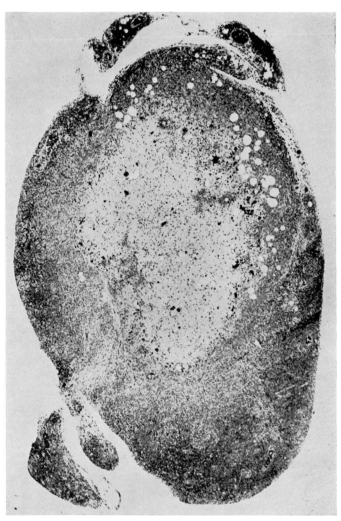

Figure IV-12. Histological preparation of a granuloma removed from the omentum. Multiple layering of viable cells may be observed around a core of foreign material mixed with necrotic macrophages and neutrophils (Athanassiades and Speirs, 1972).

grate into the granulomatous area from these blood vessels, and eosinophils, lymphocytes, and blast cells become prominent components within seven to fourteen days. Active fibroblasts are also present, and collagenic fibers gradually appear between the granuloma cells and around blood vessels. The reaction of eosinophils within the granulomas is particularly striking. They seldom contain phagocytized material and show no tendency to migrate to the medullary area, where antigen and antigenic complexes accumulate. They seem to associate primarily with mononuclear cells containing large vesicular nuclei and various amounts of rough endoplasmic reticulum with accumulated secretory material in their cisternae. In many cases, disruption of these cells occurs as a dozen or more eosinophils surround them and penetrate their cytoplasm. Lymphocytes are also associated with these rosettes but are not known to penetrate the disrupted cells. A few plasma cells are present on the seventh day, and they gradually increase in number so that, by the 28th day, they form ten or more concentric layers on the outer portion of the cell mass.

A high proportion of the granuloma cells are granulocytes, which are short-lived "end cells" incapable of division. Their sojourn in the granuloma lasts for a few hours or days, after which they are engulfed by macrophages. Other cells, especially lymphocytes and macrophages leave the granuloma, pass into the regional lymph node, and eventually spread throughout the body. Some of these cells carry information about the antigen and are "memory cells." Still other cells undergo transformation into plasma cells and secrete immunoglobulins (Athanassiades and Speirs, 1968, 1972).

Histologically, the granuloma can be subdivided into a medullary and a cortical portion (Figure IV-12). The medullary portion consists of antigenic material, necrotic cells, and scattered macrophages and neutrophils. The cortical portion, immediately surrounding the medulla, consists of layers of macrophages, with eosinophils, lymphocytes, fibroblasts, and plasma cells making up an increasingly higher proportion of the cells on the outer layer of the cortex. Adipose cells accumulate on the periphery, especially in granulomas that attach themselves to the omentum.

Usually one to four of these granulomas are formed after a single intraperitoneal inflammatory injection, and they persist in the peritoneal cavity for as long as six months after being induced.

QUANTITATIVE ESTIMATION OF CELLULAR CONTENT OF GRANULOMAS

Although granuloma formation has been the concern of many investigators in both research and clinical medicine (Athanassiades and Speirs, 1968, 1972; Spector, Lykke and Willougby, 1967; Spector and Willoughby, 1968; Warren, Domingo and Cowan, 1967; Epstein, 1967), no satisfactory procedure has been published for determining the actual number of each cell type present in granulomas at different stages of development. Since quantitative techniques had been applied to the inflammatory response, it was decided to determine the feasibility of applying similar procedures to granulomatous tissues. After a series of trials, it was found that treatment of granulomas with collagenase and pronase for one to three hours at 37° C would permit cells to be shaken free and suspended (Paul et al., 1972). Samples of the cell suspensions could be used for counting and for making smears for differential counts. The cells were found to be viable when cultured and could presumably be used for adoptive transfer experiments. An excellent correlation was noted between the results obtained with histological techniques and those obtained with cell suspensions after enzymatic treatment (Paul et al., 1972, 1973).

Subsequent experiments indicated that granulomas formed following subcutaneous injection could also be dispersed in the same manner. This was an important finding, since it justified use of the same procedures for quantitating cells at all stages, from the early inflammatory to the later chronic granulomatous responses.

Variations were found in the component-cell population, depending upon the age of the granuloma, the immunological state of the host, and the type of substance (antigenic or non-antigenic) used to induce the granuloma. Figure IV-13 shows the cellular responses of normal and primed mice to tetanus toxoid over twenty-eight days. It may be noted that, at all periods tested, the total number of cells present was highest in primed mice reinjected with specific antigen. The response in unprimed animals was similar but of lower magnitude. The response to a nonantigenic substance (aluminum phosphate) showed a different pattern, the cell count being lower than in the other two cases.

The estimated number of each kind of cell most commonly found in the developing granulomatous tissue is shown in Figure IV-13. In all groups, the neutrophil response reached a peak within twenty-four hours. The neutrophils decreased in number after the first day and remained at low levels throughout the remaining period of observation. Although eosinophils were present in all three types of granulomas induced, the highest number occurred in those animals previously primed. The eosinophils tended to persist at relatively high levels in all antigen-induced granulomas.

The mononuclear cells observed varied widely in size, shape, nuclear position, and degree of cytoplasmic basophilia. These cells consistently predominated in all three types of granulomas. Basophilic mononuclear cells and plasma cells, however, were most numerous in the granulomas induced by reinjection of specific antigen. Calculation of the number of plasma cells present at selected intervals between the fourth and the 28th days indicated that these cells increased at the rate of 2000 a day (Paul *et al.*, 1972, 1973).

The studies just described suggest that plasma cells originate from precursor blood cells attracted into an inflammatory area by antigen injection. These precursor cells (B cells), in the presence of thymic-dependent lymphocytes (T cells) and a wide variety of associated inflammatory cells, have the capacity to transform into plasma cells. The evidence at present indicates that B cells originate in the bone marrow and carry immunoglobulin (8s IgM) markers on their surface. Recent studies have demonstrated that, although these cells

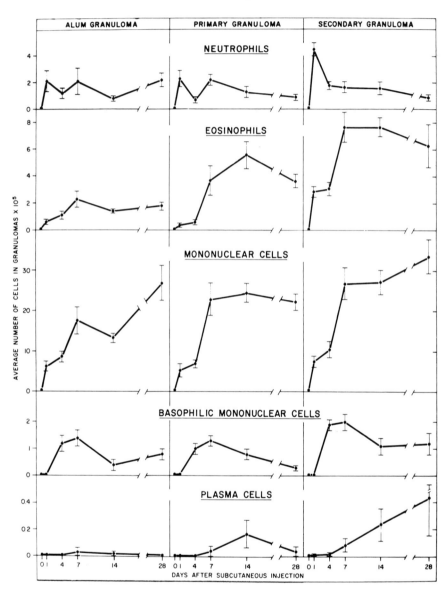

Figure IV-13. Cellular composition of granulomatous tissue at selected intervals after subcutaneous injection of aluminum phosphate or aluminum phosphate-adsorbed tetanus toxoid. Quantitation was performed after enzymatic digestion of granulomas. Smears were also made from the suspended cells to determine the number of each type of cell present (Paul, Athanassiades and Speirs, 1972).

have a paucity of cytoplasmic machinery and do not synthesize DNA, they are highly active metabolically (Uhr and Vitetta, 1973). The transformation into plasma cells seems to involve a shift in the type of immunoglobulin synthesized, a shift from an IgM to an IgG (Pierce, Asofsky and Solliday, 1973).

ROLE OF EOSINOPHILS IN THE INFLAMMATORY RESPONSE

Except in allergy and parasitic infestations, eosinophils have been generally ignored by pathologists and immunologists. Eosinophils are often overlooked or are not distinguished from neutrophils. Although their granules are very conspicuous under phase or electron microscopy, eosinophils, stained with hematoxylin and eosin and viewed under the light microscope, are usually inconspicuous against a background of connective tissue and proteinaceous material.

Eosinophils, like neutrophils, are "end cells": They have a segmented nucleus, usually bilobed in man and ring-shaped in mouse and rat. Their cytoplasm is packed with large acidophilic granules (Fig. IV-14). The granules, produced during an early stage of cell development in the bone marrow, contain a crystalloid material (presumably stored enzymes) surrounded by an arginine-rich basic protein containing acid phosphatase and peroxidase. The cytoplasm contains ribonuclease, amylsulfatase, and cathepsin.

Eosinophils are ameboid and show chemotactic activity with occasional phagocytosis (Welsh and Geer, 1959; Archer and Hirsch, 1963; Lehrer, 1971; Ishikawa, Yu and Arbesman, 1972). Unlike neutrophils, they are found only in small numbers in acute inflammation but tend to increase in number during chronic reactions induced by antigenic material. The variations in response are presumably due to differences in specific chemotactic mediators (Keller and Sorkin, 1969). Eosinophils are particularly prominent in parasitic infestations, especially in animals reinfected with the same parasite (Boyer, Basten and Beeson, 1970; Rothwell and Dineen, 1972).

Figure IV-15 illustrates the life cycle of the eosinophil. Precursor cells under specific stimulatory influences prolif-

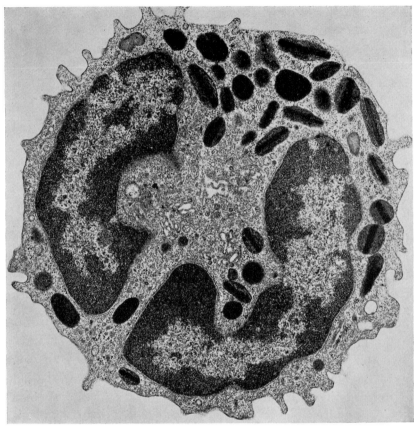

Figure IV-14. Eosinophil cell. The centrosome area of the cell is shown with portions of a Golgi apparatus. The nuclear material is highly condensed and segmented. The cytoplasm contains large granules with distinct banding.

erate and differentiate in the bone marrow. Spry (1971) demonstrated that, in the rat, eosinophils tend to accumulate in the spleen immediately after being produced in the bone marrow and prior to the time they are found in the peripheral circulation. He suggested that residence in the spleen may be a stage in the maturation of eosinophils. In any case, mature cells with preformed granules pass into the blood vessels and are distributed throughout the body, forming a consistent component of blood, lymph, and tissue fluid. They

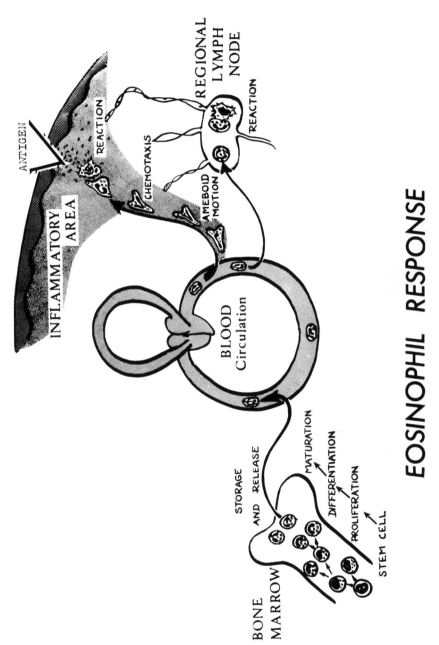

Figure IV-15. Eosinophils are produced by differentiation of precursor cells in the bone marrow. They are released into the blood where they circulate for a short time before taking part in cellular reactions either in the inflammatory area or in the regional lymph nodes. After meals containing protein, eosinophils also accumulate in large numbers in the *lamina propria* of the gut (Speirs, 1970).

are normally found in great numbers in loose connective tissue beneath the epidermis; in the *lamina propria* of the gut; in the appendix, the uterine mucosa (peaking here at the time of estrus), the lactating breast, and the lung; and in lymphatic tissues, such as lymph nodes and spleen (Rytoma, 1960; Bassett, 1962).

Two separate eosinophil responses are of special concern. The eosinophils play a minor part in all acute inflammatory reactions but a major one (usually) in chronic immunological reactions to antigen. Much of the controversy over the specificity of the eosinophil response to antigen can be explained if it is understood that, though eosinophils can be present in both types of response, the factors triggering their accumulation may be quite different (see review by Speirs, 1970).

In the acute response, a transient accumulation of extravascular eosinophils occurs within twenty-four hours. This is presumably evoked by histamine, or similar vasodilating agents, released as a result of tissue-cell contact with foreign material or of antigen-antibody reactions (Kay, 1970). The eosinophils, along with all the other blood-borne cells, leave the capillaries and venules and permeate the surrounding area. The magnitude of the eosinophil response during the acute stage is directly related to the number of eosinophils in circulation (Parish, 1972).

In the chronic response to reinjection of specific antigen, a prolonged or persisting phase occurs, in which eosinophils continue to accumulate beyond the second day and are retained in the inflammatory exudate in considerable numbers up to the seventh day. In contrast to the acute response, marked eosinopoiesis can also be demonstrated (Jenkins et al., 1972). In granulomatous tissue induced by injections of tetanus toxoid or by parasitic infestations, eosinophils may persist for many months, a reaction which appears to be related to the continued presence of antigenic components. Steele and Rack (1965) injected polystyrene beads coated with conjugates of various materials into rabbits and a guinea pig. They noted that, in contrast to uncoated beads, beads coated with antigenic conjugates induced a local accumulation of eosinophils that persisted for as long as eight months.

Eosinophils are relatively short-lived cells. Their life span in the tissues appears to be three to seven days, after which they are engulfed by macrophages. It would therefore seem that the persisting local accumulation of eosinophils must represent a continued migration of these cells into the lesion. If the antigen is neutralized by antibody, the eosinophil migration does not continue beyond the initial acute period (Speirs and Turner, 1969).

The role of antigen in these responses was demonstrated in experiments in which tritiated tetanus toxoid was used for either the priming or the challenging injection (Speirs and Speirs, 1963, 1964). After an injection of tritiated tetanus toxin neutralized with isologous antitoxin, the subjects exhibited eosinophils that were never significantly labelled above background, although the neutrophils and macrophages contained a great deal of the material. When sensitized with non-labelled tetanus toxoid and challenged with labelled tetanus toxin, the subjects exhibited many eosinophils, as well as neutrophils and macrophages, that became labelled. The labelled eosinophils were observed only after they had sufficient time to form rosettes with labelled mononuclear cells. When radioactively labelled toxin was included in a series of sensitizing injections, it was noted that the resulting labelled mononuclear cells were exquisitely sensitive on reexposure to non-labelled tetanus antigen. Rosettes of eosinophils around labelled mononuclear cells were commonly found in the inflammatory exudate.

When sensitized to diphtheria toxoid plus radioactively labelled tetanus toxin and challenged with diphtheria toxoid, the eosinophils were attracted primarily to cells not labelled. The release of chemotactic mediators may be considered a manifestation of immunity, since it occurs as a specific response to challenge. The mononuclear cell that releases the mediator must contain a component of the antigen to which it has been sensitized, as well as a component of the challenging antigen itself. Thus eosinophils are attracted to cells containing components of both the sensitizing antigen and the challenging antigen.

The reaction to specifically sensitized lymphocytes is not unique to eosinophils. It has been repeatedly demonstrated that antigen can react with sensitized lymphocytes to produce soluble mediators or lymphokines (Dumonde et al., 1969) that induce a variety of biological effects both in vivo and in vitro. These include cytotoxicity, macrophage-migration inhibition, and blastogenesis, as well as chemotaxis (David, 1971). The sensitized cells appear soon after exposure to the antigen. Atkins et al., (1972) found sensitized lymphocytes present in the regional lymph nodes by the fifth day. Upon reexposure to antigen, these lymphocytes release soluble mediators which act upon blood leukocytes. Asherson, Allison and Zembala (1972) demonstrated that sensitized cells have an increased tendency to migrate to inflammatory areas.

Since this tendency to settle in inflammatory areas followed skin grafting, contact sensitivity, and immunization, but not treatment with aluminum hydroxide, the reactions were considered to be related to cell-mediated immune responses. The experiments referred to, along with those of Turk and Polak (1968), Mackaness (1971), Koster and McGregor (1971), and Speirs and Speirs (1963 and 1964), indicate that cells stimulated during priming can move to subsequently induced inflammatory areas. If reexposed to the specific antigen, the cells release mediators which augment the inflammatory response and attract increased numbers of other cells to the inflamed area. The lesion induced is typically infiltrated by large numbers of mononuclear cells derived for the most part from the bone marrow (Lubaroff and Waksman, 1967; Bosman and Feldman, 1968). The initiation and the extent of the infiltration seem to depend upon the presence of a relatively few sensitized cells within the lesion. These sensitized cells are components of blood and lymphatic tissues and are, apparently, thymic-dependent (Waksman, Arnason and Jankovic, 1962). It has been noted, however, that, in hypersensitive reactions, in which the amount of antigen injected is too small to stimulate antibody synthesis, a third injection of antigen given

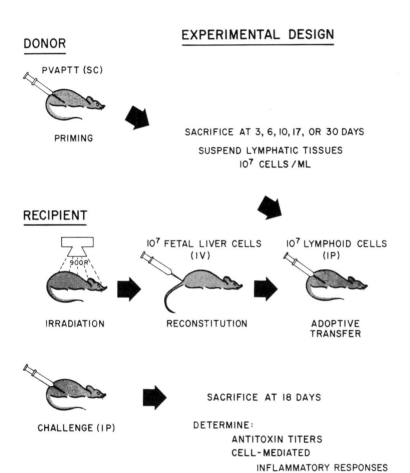

EXPERIMENTAL DESIGN

DONOR

PVAPTT (SC)

PRIMING

SACRIFICE AT 3, 6, 10, 17, OR 30 DAYS
SUSPEND LYMPHATIC TISSUES
10^7 CELLS / ML

RECIPIENT

10^7 FETAL LIVER CELLS
(IV)

10^7 LYMPHOID CELLS
(IP)

IRRADIATION

RECONSTITUTION

ADOPTIVE
TRANSFER

CHALLENGE (IP)

SACRIFICE AT 18 DAYS

DETERMINE:
ANTITOXIN TITERS
CELL-MEDIATED
INFLAMMATORY RESPONSES

Figure IV-16. Experimental Design. Adoptive transfer of lymphoid cells at selected intervals after a single priming injection of tetanus toxoid in a pertussis vaccine adjuvant. Ten million lymphoid cells are injected intraperitoneally into isogeneic mice which have been lethally irradiated and reconstituted with fetal-liver cells. The recipient mice are challenged intraperitoneally with tetanus toxoid and the cellular responses and humoral antitoxin responses noted eighteen days later. (Ponzio and Speirs, 1973).

at the site of challenge results in another massive infiltration of cells. In this, eosinophils are the major component. Arnason and Waksman (1963) named this the "retest reaction." It was specific, occurred in the absence of detectable antibody, and was inhibited by antilymphocytic serum. The retest reaction seemed to be a general phenomenon elicited at any site where a delayed type of reaction had previously been induced.

The experiments mentioned above indicate that large accumulations of eosinophils are related to the cell-mediated immune response rather than to the antibody-mediated response. This accords with the results obtained by Dineen and his coworkers, who studied the eosinophil response in infestation with the parasite *Trichostrongylus colubriformis*. These investigators noted that adoptive transfer of mesenteric lymph-node cells from immune guinea pigs resulted in bone-marrow eosinopoiesis and a local accumulation of eosinophils in the intestine of the infected recipient. The transferred sensitized lymphocytes, which were thymic-dependent, apparently underwent allergic death in the presence of the parasite and triggered the eosinophil response (Dineen, Ronai and Wagland, 1968; Rothwell and Dineen, 1972).

Recent experiments (Ponzio and Speirs, 1973) have further clarified these reactions. The experimental technique involved adoptive transfer of lymphoid cells to syngeneic irradiated animals, which were then challenged and their cellular response observed for eighteen days (Fig. IV-16). Following priming of donor mice, cells capable of transferring the capacity to induce an eosinophil response began to appear in lymphatic tissue within three to six days, and persisted for long periods thereafter (Fig. IV-17). These lymphoid cells, called "memory cells," did not induce an eosinophil response unless the recipient animal was reexposed to the specific antigen. The response was not obtained with lymphoid cells taken from normal mice or mice primed with an antigen different from that used for the challenge. The induction of these memory cells occurred prior to the time of antitoxin production and prior to the formation of cells capable of transferring secondary humoral antitoxin production. Since the memory cells were not found in mice de-

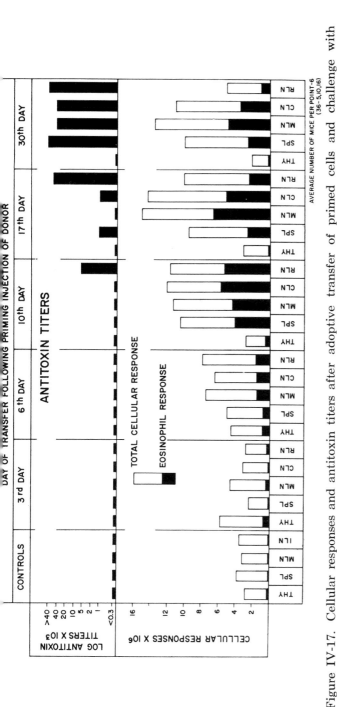

Figure IV-17. Cellular responses and antitoxin titers after adoptive transfer of primed cells and challenge with tetanus toxoid. Cells capable of augmenting the cellular response can be detected by adoptive transfer between three and six days after priming. By the tenth day and thereafter, they are present in all lymphatic tissues transferred, except the thymus. Transfer of the capacity to mount a secondary humoral antitoxin response is not detectable at the end of the third day or the sixth. Transfer of regional lymph-node cells on the tenth day induces antitoxin production. Cells of other lymph nodes and spleen do not attain this capacity until the seventeenth day after priming (Ponzio and Speirs, 1973). Abbreviations. THY—Thymus; SPL—Spleen; MLN—Mesenteric Lymph Node; ILN—Inguinal Lymph Node; RLN—Regional Lymph Node (Inguinal); CLN—Contralateral Lymph Node (Inguinal).

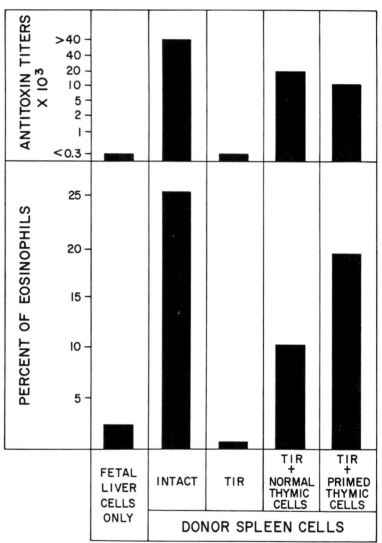

AVERAGE NUMBER OF MICE PER POINT-4

(36-1)

Figure IV-18. Eosinophil and antitoxin titers in TIR (thymic-depleted) mice and TIR mice pretreated with normal or primed thymic cells. The presence of thymic-dependent cells is essential for the induction of memory cells to both secondary humoral and eosinophil response to tetanus toxoid (Ponzio and Speirs, 1973).

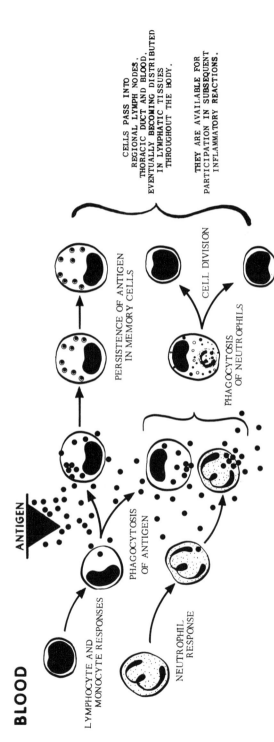

Figure IV-19. Primary response. Cellular responses to a primary injection of antigen. Neutrophils, monocytes, and lymphocytes leave the blood vessels to make up the chief cellular components of the inflammatory exudate. Antigenic fragments persist as cytoplasmic components of both lymphocytes and macrophages and are carried to the regional lymph nodes and eventually to lymphatic tissues throughout the body. These cells are referred to as memory cells, since they can recognize and react to reexposure of the specific antigen.

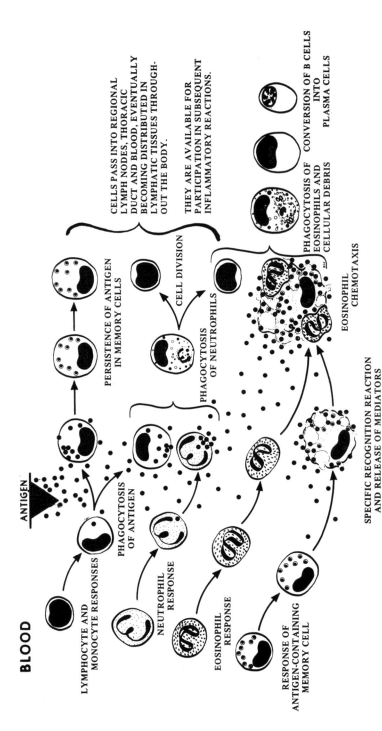

ANAMNESTIC RESPONSE

BLOOD

ANTIGEN

LYMPHOCYTE AND MONOCYTE RESPONSES

PHAGOCYTOSIS OF ANTIGEN

NEUTROPHIL RESPONSE

EOSINOPHIL RESPONSE

RESPONSE OF ANTIGEN-CONTAINING MEMORY CELL

SPECIFIC RECOGNITION REACTION AND RELEASE OF MEDIATORS

PERSISTENCE OF ANTIGEN IN MEMORY CELLS

CELL DIVISION

PHAGOCYTOSIS OF NEUTROPHILS

CELLS PASS INTO REGIONAL LYMPH NODES, THORACIC DUCT AND BLOOD, EVENTUALLY BECOMING DISTRIBUTED IN LYMPHATIC TISSUES THROUGH-OUT THE BODY.

THEY ARE AVAILABLE FOR PARTICIPATION IN SUBSEQUENT INFLAMMATORY REACTIONS.

PHAGOCYTOSIS OF EOSINOPHILS AND CELLULAR DEBRIS

EOSINOPHIL CHEMOTAXIS

CONVERSION OF B CELLS INTO PLASMA CELLS

CELLULAR RESPONSE TO ANTIGEN

pleted of thymic cells by thymectomy, irradiation, and reconstitution with fetal-liver cells (TIR mice), it was concluded
that they must be thymic-dependent. Restoration of the capacity of the donor animals to produce memory cells occurred
when a suspension of thymic cells was given them one week
before priming (Fig. IV-18). A similar requirement for thymic
lymphocytes in the induction of local and systemic eosinophil
responses has also been demonstrated by Walls *et al.* (1971)
and Boyer, Basten and Beeson (1970).

The role of the eosinophil has not been fully elucidated.
It has been shown to be involved in immunological responses,
especially when the antigen persists, as in chronic infections,
or reenters the body at some subsequent period. Eosinophils
are chemotactically attracted to specific memory cells containing components of both the priming antigen and the challenging antigen. They are later engulfed by macrophages just
before plasma-cell formation. Macrophages are essential to
the T- and B-cell collaboration leading to antibody formation
(Feldmann, 1972). Furthermore, it has been shown that B cells
first bind themselves to macrophages (Schmidtke and Unanue,
1971) and then undergo mitosis and differentiation into plasma
cells (Nossal and Makela, 1962, Bosman and Feldmann, 1968;
Mosier, 1969). Since the eosinophil is involved both with
memory cells and with macrophages, it may act as helper
or intermediary in carrying immunological information (possibly in the form of RNA) to the macrophages, which in turn
pass it along to cells that subsequently produce antibody
(Speirs, 1970, 1971).

←————————————————————————————————

Figure IV-20. Cellular responses to a challenging injection of antigen.
The inflammatory reaction begins in the same manner as in the primary response, with neutrophils, lymphocytes, and monocytes playing
the predominant roles. Memory cells containing components of antigen from earlier injection, however, take part in the reaction. These
cells recognize the antigen and become swollen and vacuolated. They
release mediators which augment the inflammatory response by attracting additional mononuclear cells and eosinophils to the inflamed
area. Information seems to be passed from the memory cells to cells
capable of transforming themselves into plasma cells.

Two diagrams sum up the role of various cells in the immunological response to tetanus toxoid. Figure IV-19 indicates the cellular reactions most typical of the primary response, monocytes and neutrophils playing the predominant role. Eosinophils play a very minor role, the number taking part being determined primarily by the number in circulation and the intensity of the stimulation. As granulocytes are gradually consumed during the inflammatory response, mononuclear cells begin to predominate. These subsequently leave the inflammatory or granulomatous areas and are carried by a stream of fluid to the lymphatics and the regional lymph node; eventually, they make their way to the thoracic duct and the blood vessels. Some of these cells, because they carry immunological information, are referred to as memory cells. The memory cells, which are antigen-sensitive, are temporarily stored in lymphatic tissue and become a component of subsequent inflammatory exudates. When reexposed to the specific antigen, they initiate two different reactions (Fig. IV-20). First, mediators are released that augment the cellular reactions specifically attracting eosinophils and additional mononuclear cells to the inflammatory area. Second, memory cells, in the presence of eosinophils and macrophages, convert B cells into plasma cells that produce and secrete immunoglobulins.

Thus these inflammatory and granulomatous reactions involve a sequential pattern of local and systemic cellular responses. Every phase involves the coordinated activity of millions of cells, each cell responding to changes in its microenvironment in an individualistic manner. As a result of these combined reactions, a state of tolerance, immunity, or hypersensitivity is determined within the host.

REFERENCES

Archer, G. T., Hirsch, J. G.: Motion-picture studies on degranulation of horse eosinophils during phagocytosis. *J Exp Med, 118:* 287, 1963.

Arnason, B. G., Waksman, B. H.: The retest reaction in delayed hypersensitivity. *Lab Invest, 12:* 737–47, 1963.

Asherson, G. L., Allison, A. C., and Zembala, M.: Production of delayed hypersensitivity by antigen associated with peritoneal-exudate cells and the effect of pretreatment with Freund's complete adjuvant. *Immunology, 22:* 465–473, 1972.

Athanassiades, T. J., and Speirs, R. S.: Formation of antigen-induced granulomas containing plasma cells: a light- and electron-microscopic study. *J Reticuloendothel Soc, 5:* 485–97, 1968.

Athanassiades, T. J., and Speirs, R. S.: Granuloma induction in the peritoneal cavity. A model for the study of inflammation and plasmacytopoiesis in nonlymphatic organs. *J Reticuloendothel Soc, 11:* 60–76, 1972.

Atkins, E., Feldman, J. D., Francis, L., Hursh, E.: Studies on the mechanism of fever accompanying delayed hypersensitivity. *J Exp Med, 135:* 1113, 1972.

Bassett, E. G.: Infiltration of eosinophils into the modified connective tissue of oestrous and pregnant animals. *Nature, 194:* 1259, 1962.

Bosman, C., and Feldman, J. D.: Cytology of immunologic memory—a morphologic study of lymphoid cells during the anamnestic response. *J Exp Med, 125:* 293, 1968.

Boyer, M. H., Basten, A., Beeson, P. B.: Mechanism of Eosinophilia III. Suppression of eosinophilia by agents known to modify immune responses. *Blood, 36:* 458, 1970.

David, J. R.: Mediators produced by sensitized lymphocytes. *Fed Proc, 30:* 1730–35, 1971.

Day, R. P.: Eosinophil-cell separation from human peripheral blood. *Immunology, 18:* 955, 1970.

Dineen, J. K., Ronai, P. M., and Wagland, B. M.: The cellular transfer of immunity to *trichostrongylus colubriformis* in an isogeneic strain of guinea pig. IV. The localization of immune lymphocytes in small intestine in infected and noninfected guinea pigs. *Immunology, 16:* 671, 1968.

Dumonde, D. C., Wolstencroft, R. A., Panayi, G. S., Matthew, M., Morley, J., and Howson, W. T.: "Lymphokines": nonantibody mediators of cellular immunity generated by lymphocyte activation. *Nature, 224:* 38–42, 1969.

Epstein, W. L.: Granulomatous hypersensitivity. *Progress in Allergy, 11:* 36–88, 1967.

Feldmann, M.: Cell interactions in the immune response *in vitro.* II. The requirement for macrophages in lymphoid-cell collaboration. *J Exp Med, 135:* 1049–58, 1972.

Ishikawa, T., Yu, M. C., and Arbesman, C. E.: Electron-microscopic demonstration of phagocytosis of *Candida albicans* by human eosinophilic leukocytes. *J Allergy Clin Immunol, 50:* 183, 1972.

Jenkins, V. K., Trentin, J. J., Speirs, R. S., and McGarry, M. P.: Hemopoietic colony studies. VI. Increased eosinophil-containing colonies by antigen pretreatment of irradiated mice reconstituted with bone-marrow cells. *J Cell Physiol, 79:* 413, 1972.

Kay, A. B.: Studies on eosinophil-leucocyte migration. 1. Eosinophil and neutrophil accumulation following antigen-antibody reactions in guinea pig skin. *Clin Exp Immunol, 6:* 75, 1970.

Keller, H. U., and Sorkin, E.: Studies on chemotaxis. XIII. Differences in the chemotactic response of neutrophil and eosinophil polymorphonuclear leucocytes. *Int Arch Allergy Appl Immunol, 35:* 279, 1969.

Koster, F. T., and McGregor, D. D.: The mediator of cellular immunity. III. Lymphocyte traffic from the blood into the inflamed peritoneal cavity. *J Exp Med, 133:* 864, 1971.

Lehrer, R. I.: Measurement of candidacidal activity of specific leukocyte types in mixed cell populations. II. Normal and chronic granulomatous-disease eosinophils. *Infect Immun, 3:* 800, 1971.

Lubaroff, D. M., and Waksman, B. H.: Delayed hypersensitivity: bone marrow as the source of cells in delayed skin reactions. *Science, 157:* 322, 1967.

McGarry, M. P., Speirs, R. S., Jenkins, V. K., and Trentin, J. J.: Lymphoid cell dependence of eosinophil response to antigen. *J Exp Med, 134:* 801–814, 1971.

Mackaness, G. B.: Resistance to intracellular infection. *J Infect Dis, 123:* 439–45, 1971.

Mann, P. R.: An electron-microscope study of the relations between mast cells and eosinophil leucocytes. *J Pathol, 98:* 183–186, 1969.

Miller, H. R. P., and Avrameas, S.: Association between macrophages and specific antibody-producing cells. *Nature [New Biol], 229:* 184, 1971.

Mosier, D. E.: Cell interactions in the primary immune response *in vitro:* a requirement for specific cell clusters. *J Exp Med, 129:* 351–63, 1969.

Nossal, G. J. V., and Makela, O.: Autoradiographic studies on the immune response. *J Exp Med, 115:* 209–230, 1962.

Parish, W. E.: Eosinophilia. II. Cutaneous eosinophilia in guinea pigs mediated by passive anaphylaxis with IgGI or Reagin and antigen-antibody complexes: its relation to neutrophils and mast cells. *Immunology, 23:* 19, 1972.

Paul, S. D., Athanassiades, T. J., and Speirs, R. S.: A quantitative procedure for the study of cells in experimentally induced granulomas. *Proc Soc Exp Biol Med, 139:* 1090, 1972.

Paul, S. D., Athanassiades, T. J., and Speirs, R. S.: The immunosuppressive effect of dactinomycin on experimentally induced granulomas. *Proc Soc Exp Biol Med, 143:* 222–229, 1973.

Pierce, C. W., Asofsky, R., and Solliday, S. M.: Immunoglobulin receptors on B lymphocytes: shift in immunoglobulin class during immune responses. *Fed Proc, 32:* 41–43, 1973.

Ponzio, N. M., and Speirs, R. S.: Lymphoid dependence of eosinophil response to antigen. III. Comparison of the rate of appearance of two types of memory cell in various lymphoid tissues at different times after priming. *J Immunol, 110:* 6, 1973.

Rothwell, T. L. W., and Dineen, J. K.: Cellular reactions in guinea pigs following primary and challenge infection with *Trichostrongylus colubriformis*, with special reference to the roles played by eosinophils and basophils in rejection of the parasite. *Immunology, 22:* 733, 1972.

Rytoma, T.: Organ distribution and histochemical properties of eosinophil granulocytes in rat. *Acta Pathol et Microbiol Scand Suppl, 140:* 1960, v. 50.

Schmidtke, J., and Unanue, E. R.: Interaction of macrophages and lymphocytes with surface immunoglobulin. *Nature, 233:* 84–6, 1971.

Spector, W. G., and Willoughby, D. A.: The origin of mononuclear cells in chronic inflammation and tuberculin reactions in the rat. *J Pathol Bact, 96:* 389–99, 1968.

Spector, W. G., Lykke, A. W. J., and Willoughby, D. A.: A quantitative study of leucocyte emigration in chronic inflammatory granulomata. *J Pathol Bact, 93:* 101–107, 1967.

Speirs, R. S.: Advances in the knowledge of the eosinophil in relation to antibody formation, *Annals of the New York Academy of Science, 73:* 283–306, 1958.

Speirs, R. S.: Distribution of tritiated tetanus toxin following an intraperitoneal injection in immunized and nonimmunized mice. In *Tritium in the Physical and Biological Sciences* 1962, vol. VII, pp. 419–28.

Speirs, R. S.: Function of leukocytes in inflammation and immunity. In Gordon, A. S. (Ed.): Regulation of Hematopoiesis. New York, Appleton, 1970.

Speirs, R. S.: Multiple cellular and subcellular responses to antigen. Literature Review and Hypothesis of Inflammation. *Immunochemistry, 8:* 665–689, 1971.

Speirs, R. S.: Relation of eosinophils to antibody formation. *J Reticuloenidothel Soc bull, 3:* 19–22, 1957.

Speirs, R. S., and Dreisbach, M.: Quantitative studies of the cellular responses to antigen injections in normal mice. *Blood, 11:* 44–55, 1956.

Speirs, R. S., and Osada, Y.: Chemotactic activity and phagocytosis of eosinophils. *Proc Soc Exp Biol Med, 109:* 929–932, 1962.

Speirs, R. S., and Speirs, E. E.: Cellular localization of radioactive antigen in immunized and nonimmunized mice. *J Immunol, 90:* 561–75, 1963.

Speirs, R. S., and Speirs, E. E.: Cellular reactions to reinjection of antigen. *J Immunol, 92:* 540–49, 1964.

Speirs, R. S., and Turner, M. X.: The eosinophil response to toxoids and its inhibition by antitoxin. *Blood, 34:* 320–330, 1969.

Speirs, R. S., and Wenck, U.: Eosinophil response to toxoids in actively and passively immunized mice. *Proc Soc Exp Biol Med, 90:* 571–74, 1955.

Speirs, R. S., Jansen, V., Speirs, E. E., Osada, S., and Dienes, L.: Use of tritiated thymidine to study the origin and fate of inflammatory cells. In *Tritium in the Physical and Biological Sciences.* 1962, vol. VII, pp. 301–26.

Speirs, R. S., Speirs, E. E., and Jansen, V.: A quantitative approach to the study of inflammatory cells. *Proc Soc Exp Biol Med, 106:* 248–251, 1961.

Spry, C. J. F.: Mechanism of eosinophilia. V. Kinetics of normal and accelerated eosinopoiesis. *Cell Tissue Kinet, 4:* 351–364, 1971.

Spry, C. J. F.: The origin kinetics and distribution of large lymphocytes from the thoracic duct of rats with trichinosis. *Immunology, 22:* 663–75, 1972.

Steele, A. S. V., and Rack, J. H.: Cellular reaction to polystyrene-protein conjugates. *J. Pathol Bact, 89:* 703, 1965.

Turk, J. L., and Polack, L.: A comparison of the effect of anti-lymph-node serum and anti-granulocyte serum on local passive transfer of the tuberculin reaction and the normal lymphocyte reaction. *Int Arch Allergy Appl Immunol, 34:* 105–118, 1968.

Turner, M. X., Speirs, R. S., and McLaughlin, J.: Effect of Primary Injection Site upon cellular and Antitoxin Responses to Subsequent Challenging Injections. *Proceedings of the Society for Experimental Biology and Medicine, 129:* 738–743, 1968.

Uhr, J. W., and Vitetta, E. S.: Synthesis, biochemistry, and dynamics of cell-surface immunoglobulin on lymphocytes. *Fed Proc, 32:* 35–40, 1973.

Waksman, B. H., Arnason, B. G., and Jankovic, B. D.: Role of the thymus in immune reactions in rats. III. Changes in the lymphoid organs of thymectomized rats. *J Exp Med, 116:* 187, 1962.

Walls, R. S., Basten, A., Leuchars, E., and Davies, A. J. S.: Mechanism for eosinophilic and neutrophilic leucocytes. *Br Med J, 3:* 157, 1971.

Warren, K. S., Domingo, E. O., and Cowan, R. B. T.: Granuloma formation around schistosome eggs as a manifestation of delayed hypersensitivity. *Am J Pathol, 51:* 735, 1967.

Welsh, R. A., Geer, J. C.: Phagocytosis of mast-cell granules by the eosinophilic leukocyte in the rat. *Am J Pathol, 35:* 103–108, 1959.

CHAPTER V

THE MACROPHAGE

W. G. SPECTOR and D. A. WILLOUGHBY

A CHRONIC INFLAMMATORY INFILTRATE, especially if granulomatous, consists of cells derived from three lines— the mononuclear phagocyte, the lymphoid, and the fibroblast. In addition, there are the representatives of the granulocytic series, especially eosinophils.

Fibroblasts produce collagen, ground substance, and, by mitotic division, more fibroblasts. Lymphoid cells appear as lymphocytes, plasma cells, or immunoblasts. Mononuclear phagocytes are seen as macrophages, epithelioid cells, or giant cells. The three cell lines are distinct and are incapable of transformation from one to another. Although, at certain stages of the disease, lymphocytes, fibroblasts, or granulocytes may seem to be dominant, the true architectural unit of chronic inflammation is almost always the macrophage and its derivatives, the epithelioid cell and the giant cell.

The Origin of Inflammatory Macrophages

The macrophages of the inflammatory response have been variously supposed to originate from circulating monocytes, lymphocytes, or connective-tissue cells. Early work based on sequential study of cells containing a cytoplasmic-carbon marker demonstrated the entry of monocytes into inflamed areas and their subsequent transformation into macrophages (Ebert and Florey, 1939). These studies, however, left unanswered the problem of how many of the inflammatory macrophages had that derivation. The

93

introduction of tritiated thymidine (3HT) made it possible to say that at least most of the mononuclear cells
making up an inflammatory exudate were derived from the
circulation rather than formed *in situ* (Cronkite *et al.*, 1960;
Kosunen *et al.*, 1963). Spector, Walters and Willoughby
(1965) and Volkman and Gowans (1965a), using 3HT and
carbon and 3HT alone, respectively, demonstrated that it was
in fact the monocyte in the circulation that was the major
precursor of inflammatory macrophages, at least in certain
simple types of injury. Volkman and Gowans (1965b) showed
also that the macrophage precursor in question was undoubt-
edly of bone-marrow origin. Spector and Willoughby (1968)
investigated inflammation of a more complex type—the granulomata induced by incomplete Freund adjuvant. In rats whose
bone marrow and lymphoid tissue had been destroyed by X
irradiation, there was a virtual absence of macrophages
in such granulomata, unless bone-marrow cells were given
as therapy intravenously. Similar intravenous injection of
lymph node or thymus cells failed to provide a source of
macrophages. Having entered the area of inflammation and
become macrophages, the marrow cells underwent further transformation to epithelioid and giant cells and perithelial cells.
One result of these observations was to lessen the investigators'
interest in the relative roles of connective tissue and circulating cells in macrophage genesis, since both types of precursor
seemed to be of marrow origin. It should be added that recent
results make it seem very unlikely that fibroblasts or vascular
endothelium are derived from macrophages or macrophage precursors (Giroud, Spector and Willoughby, 1970; Ross, Everett
and Tyler, 1969).

    In spite of certain morphological evidence suggesting that
lymphocytes might be the progenitors of inflammatory
macrophages, the authors of this chapter have never found
lymphocytes to be the initial source of macrophages that
colonize an inflammatory reaction. They have, however,
seen lymphocytes enter established reactions induced some
weeks earlier by complete Freund adjuvant. Reactions of
this type contain lymphoid foci apparently derived from

bone-marrow lymphopoietic precursors. It may therefore be that the entry of circulating lymphocytes into such established lesions represents recirculation of cells through what could be regarded as an ectopic lymph node.

Similar methods have been used to study the derivation of the mononuclear cells constituting a tuberculin reaction in rats (Spector and Willoughby, 1968). Once again it was observed that only marrow cells could give rise to the inflammatory mononuclears, in spite of the lymphocytic appearance of the cells in question. Even marrow cells from unsensitized donors could give rise to a tuberculin reaction, provided that lymphocytes from sensitized donors were given simultaneously.

Thus, in various types of reaction, marrow cells have been shown to provide classical macrophages, cells with the morphological appearance of lymphocytes and connective-tissue histiocytes. In other observations (Giroud, Spector and Willoughby, 1970), marrow cells were found to be responsible for the mononuclear-cell reaction that accompanies the rejection of skin allografts in mice, although the addition of lymphocytes to the marrow inoculum accelerated the allograft rejection in the irradiated recipients.

The Fate of Inflammatory Macrophages

Infiltration of inflamed tissues by macrophages may be transient or persistent, depending on the cause of the injury. In acute inflammation, the macrophages disappear within a few days, owing to the death of the cells or to their migration to other areas or loss of them by way of the lymphatics. In chronic inflammation, persistence of macrophages could be due to mitotic division, sustained recruitment from the bone marrow, or longevity of the cells in the tissues. We have in fact evidence of all three mechanisms.

The Proliferation of Macrophages

Whether or not inflammatory macrophages exhibit premitotic synthesis of DNA has been the subject of some debate. Volkman and Gowans (1965a), studying macrophages adherent to glass coverslips inserted subcutaneously, found little DNA synthesis at the end of twenty-four or forty-eight hours. On the other hand, Spector and Lykke (1966), using similar pulse labelling with 3HT, found extensive DNA synthesis in connective-tissue macrophages in inflammatory reactions of forty-eight hours' duration; in other types of injury, similar cells showed uptake of a pulse of 3HT as early as twenty-four hours after injury (Spector, Heesom and Stevens, 1968). A possible explanation of this discrepancy came first from the observation of Spector and Lykke that uptake of 3HT occurred in the perivascular macrophages earlier than in the diffuse exudate cells. It seemed possible that glass coverslips might somehow select these latter non-DNA-synthesizing cells. Ryan and Spector (1970) therefore inserted glass coverslips subcutaneously and traced the pattern of DNA synthesis in, respectively, the macrophages of the connective tissue and the macrophages adhering to the coverslips. In the connective-tissue macrophages, synthesis of nuclear DNA was extensive as early as four hours after injury and reached its peak in two or three days; this confirmed the results of Spector and Lykke. On the other hand, macrophages adhering to the subcutaneous coverslips showed virtually no uptake of a pulse of 3HT for the first three days; and this confirmed the findings of Volkman and Gowans. On the fourth day, however, the coverslip macrophages began to exhibit extensive DNA synthesis, the process coinciding with a decline in the percentage of connective-tissue macrophages taking up a pulse of 3HT. It is therefore plain that the discrepancies observed in DNA synthesis in the nuclei of inflammatory macrophages were due very largely to differences in sampling methods.

Giant cells were seen on the coverslips after the first few days had elapsed, but in lesions two or three weeks old, the nuclei of the giant cells were never observed to take up a pulse of 3HT. After two or three weeks, however, heavy nuclear labelling was seen, thus disproving the widely held view that DNA synthesis did not occur in the nuclei of inflammatory giant cells. Labelling occurred *in vivo* and *in vitro* and was sufficiently heavy to indicate that it was premitotic. In mice as opposed to rats, DNA synthesis began in inflammatory giant cells at a somewhat earlier stage; and, in mice especially, the DNA synthesis was frequently synchronous, every nucleus in the cell becoming labelled simultaneously. A similar phenomenon was seen in rats but less frequently.

It is plain that a number of differences exist between the macrophages in early reactions to implanted coverships and those of later reactions. A further variation noted was that, when macrophages from such reactions were teased out and induced to adhere to glass coverslips and the coverslips incubated for two hours in the presence of 3HT, cells from seven-day-old reactions incorporated the isotope into their own nuclear DNA, whereas those from day-old lesions failed to do so, though tissue sections taken at both time intervals showed many labelled cells. Thus the DNA-synthesizing macrophages of early lesions cannot be physically removed from the reaction, whereas those of later lesions can be. It was possible to exclude artefacts resulting from selective adhesion to glass, since similar results were obtained when smears were made of samples of all cells teased out of the lesion. In early reactions, incorporation of 3HT is largely confined to perivascular macrophages, and it may be that the situation of these cells in close association with connective-tissue fibrils in perivascular compartment makes their removal difficult.

The simplest way to explain these results is to suggest that macrophages newly arrived from the circulation undergo one spontaneous burst of DNA synthesis and, during it, cannot be detached from their surroundings. After this mitotic cycle, they become refractory to further DNA synthesis for some time and then undergo delayed and possibly sustained DNA synthesis. It is cells in this latter phase that adhere to the coverslip in the experiment described above and that can be teased out of seven-day-old coverslip reactions and shown to undergo DNA synthesis *in vitro.* Such sustained premitotic and mitotic activity could result from the release of mitogenic factors—e.g., from damaged cells. Sequential studies have shown that at least some of the DNA-synthesizing macrophages in the perivascular compartment subsequently migrate and adhere to the coverslips.

These differences could be the result of properties intrinsic to the macrophages or to changes in their environment. In an attempt to resolve this problem, coverslips containing adherent macrophages were transferred from one-day-old lesions to the site of seven-day-old lesions and *vice versa*. When the cells were tested for ability to take up a pulse of 3HT, it was found that 24-hour-old coverslip macrophages failed to synthesize DNA when transferred to a seven-day-old pocket and that seven-day-old coverslip macrophages ceased to take up the isotope when moved to a 24-hour-old pocket. It seems from this result, therefore, that something in the environment of 24-hour-old reactions inhibits DNA synthesis in macrophages but that, even if this factor were absent, coverslip macrophages of that age would be unable to enter the mitotic cycle. In contrast to their behavior when transferred to 24-hour-reactions, seven-day-old coverslip macrophages continued to synthesize DNA for at least six days when maintained in tissue culture *in vitro*, thus establishing their viability after removal from their environment. On the other hand, 24-hour-old coverslip macrophages showed no DNA synthesis when similarly cultured for six days; this emphasizes the intrinsic nature of the incapacity of these cells to undergo mitosis.

In view of the known variability in the rates at which chronic inflammatory lesions of different types are replenished by cells from the circulation (Ryan and Spector, 1969), it was clearly important to determine to what extent the proliferation of coverslip macrophages was self-perpetuating, as opposed to being dependent upon renewal by fresh recruits from the bone marrow. This was studied in rats bearing subcutaneous coverslips; the animals were subjected either to irradiation of the entire body, except for the subcutaneous tissue containing the coverslip, or to irradiation of the coverslip area only (Ryan and Spector, 1970). In this way, destruction was achieved of either the bone marrow or the mitotic potential of the cells in the region of the in-

serted coverslip. It was found that, in rats in which only
the bone marrow was destroyed, the number of macrophages on the coverslips, as well as the proportion syn-
thesizing DNA, fell steeply, indicating that this cell population is heavily dependent upon daily recruitment from
the bone marrow to maintain both its numbers and its
mitotic potential. The perivascular macrophages, many of
which were, of course, destined to adhere to the coverslip, showed a similar decline. The values obtained indicated that the average period a macrophage spent on a
coverslip was from one to three days, although for some macrophages that period may have been much longer. The
results also suggested that most of the macrophages underwent only one or perhaps two mitotic cycles before
becoming detached. Conversely, irradiation of the site
of coverslip implantation with the marrow left intact had
a minimal effect on the number or the mitotic activity
of macrophages on the coverslip or in the surrounding tissues. This result confirms the importance of a fresh daily
supply of cells from the bone marrow. When these experiments were repeated with coverslip lesions of increasing
age, similar results were obtained, but it was found that
dependence upon recruitment from the bone marrow fell with
maturation of the lesion. The experiments also confirmed the
fact that perivascular macrophages synthesize DNA shortly
after their arrival from the circulation, since there was a particularly steep fall in the uptake of 3HT by those cells after
destruction of the bone marrow by X rays (Ryan and Spector,
1970).

In the preceding discussion, the assumption has been that
nuclear DNA synthesis, as demonstrated by uptake of 3HT,
is synonymous with mitotic activity. What follows strengthens
this assumption: Monocytes were obtained from rat blood with
the aid of sedimentation in 3% gelatin and made to adhere to
glass coverslips, these being vigorously washed to remove non-
adherent cells. Granulocytes stuck to the glass but only for a
few hours. The coverslips, which thus bore small numbers of
monocytes in pure culture, were inserted subcutaneously into

rats previously subjected to whole-body irradiation to destroy any source of macrophages other than the implanted donor monocytes. At the end of forty-eight hours, the sparse initial collection of monocytes had proliferated so that the coverslip was covered with a continuous sheet of macrophages showing extensive DNA synthesis as described above. The clean coverslips, free from adherent monocytes, inserted as controls in the contralateral flanks of the same rats, were found to be devoid of cells when examined at the end of forty-eight hours (Ryan and Spector, 1970). This experiment seems to show conclusively that inflammatory macrophages not only synthesize DNA but are capable also of true mitotic proliferation with net increase in cell numbers. The experiment also offers a further demonstration of the origin of macrophages from monocytes.

It is of interest that the results of van Furth and Cohn (1968) should show that blood monocytes cultured *in vitro* have very low rates of DNA synthesis. The results of the experiment just described stress the importance of environment in determining whether macrophages enter the mitotic cycle.

The influence of environment on macrophage kinetics is shown even more strikingly by other experiments (Ryan and Spector, 1970) in which mouse and rat peritoneal macrophages were made to adhere to coverslips and were then implanted subcutaneously into hosts whose bone marrow had been destroyed by X rays. The peritoneal macrophages behaved in the same fashion as blood monocytes: The cells on the coverslips increased in number and showed heavy DNA synthesis throughout the week that followed implantation. In mice, the peak level, when 10 percent of the macrophages incorporated a pulse of 3HT, was observed at the end of two days, the cells then maintaining a 4 percent level of labelling for seven days. As is the case of monocytes, this result contrasts sharply with the behavior of peritoneal cells cultured *in vitro* in the presence of 3HT. In this system, DNA synthesis virtually ceases after twenty-four hours and even then seldom exceeds 1 percent. It will be apparent that peritoneal macrophages implanted subcutaneously differ in their behavior not only from the same cells cultured *in vitro* but also from 24-hour-old inflammatory macrophages; the peritoneal cells synthesize DNA immediately after implantation. Peritoneal macrophages also fail to resemble seven-day-old inflammatory macrophages in that they do not synthesize DNA for any length of time *in vitro*.

Long-Lived Macrophages

DNA synthesis in inflammatory macrophages is plainly very prevalent in chronic inflammatory granulomata. It was therefore surprising to find that, in reactions to certain synthetic polymers, DNA-synthesis rates among the participating macrophages were very low (Spector, Heesom and Stevens, 1968). This observation, meaningless at first, took on significance when the results of pulse labelling with 3HT in rats with carrageenan-induced granulomata were studied. Carrageenan is a relatively inert polysaccharide (digested in the body with great difficulty) that produces large and persistent accumulations of macrophages on injection. In the lesions that lasted for more than a week or two, the macrophages showed a much lower rate of DNA synthesis than would have been predicted. DNA synthesis as measured by uptake of a pulse of 3HT is, of course, one index of macrophage turnover in granulomata. Another index is the rate of disappearance of macrophages previously labelled with 3HT *in vivo* before the lesion was induced, together with the parallel decline in average nuclear-grain count. Granulomatous lesions induced by intradermal injection of Freund adjuvant or *B. pertussis* vaccine show a rapid fall in the percentage of such labelled cells as well as in their nuclear-grain count (Ryan and Spector, 1969; Spector and Lykke, 1966). The observed drop in these values is the result of mitotic proliferation with dilution of isotope, dilution of labelled cells by entry of fresh unlabelled cells from the circulation, and death of labelled cells.

Carrageenan granulomata, therefore, in spite of their large size and persistent nature, differ from similar types of reaction induced by other irritants; the rate of disappearance of labelled macrophages is very much slower and the rate of DNA synthesis, as judged by a single pulse of 3HT, is very much lower. These observations raise the possibility that the carrageenan reaction may contain a high proportion of long-lived macro-phages. That such long-lived macrophages exist has been postulated for many years, particularly by observers working with rabbit-ear chambers (Cliff, 1966; Ebert and Florey, 1939). The authors of this chapter excluded the possibility that the macrophages of the carrageenan reaction were moribund or dead by perfusing the lesions *in vivo* with tritiated uridine, thus detecting synthesis of RNA in the suspect cells. Since the macrophages were alive, were dividing at a low rate, and contained the labelled nuclear DNA with which they had originally arrived in the lesion weeks or months earlier, it had to be concluded that the carrageenan reaction is composed to a large extent of long-lived macrophages (Ryan and Spector, 1969; Spector and Ryan, 1969).

The possibility was apparent that such cells might be found in other types of chronic inflammation. Since the injec-tion of *B. pertussis* vaccine produces a lesion with a particularly rapid turnover of macrophages, two-day-old lesions so pro-duced in rats were pulse-labelled with 3HT on four consecutive days. Some of the rats received a second course of 3HT when the granulomata were four weeks old. As might be expected, only a very small number of tritium-labelled cells were found when the reactions were examined at the end of five and eight weeks respectively. Since the body contained no reservoir of labelled cells or of free label, it seems very likely that such tritiated macrophages as were evident in the *B. pertussis* le-sions were indeed of the long-lived variety. With time the *B. pertussis* granuloma dwindles in size; and, during this pro-cess, the percentage of labelled macrophages increases, as does the number of such cells containing phagocytosed *B. pertussis* organisms (Ryan and Spector, 1970). It would therefore seem possible that, in a granuloma, with a high cell turnover, a process of natural selection may occur in the macrophage pop-ulation, this resulting in gradual preponderance of long-lived cells. The process by which the long-lived macrophages come eventually to sequester most of the remaining irritant is an extremely slow one and is therefore probably random rather than selective. This sequestration may occur (1) because the irritant is no longer toxic to macrophages and the cells are therefore permitted to express an innate tendency to long life or (2) because the long-lived cells in question possess the additional property of resistance to damage by the irritant.

Recruitment from Circulating Macrophage Precursors

Direct measurement of the rate of emigration of monocytes from the circulation to granulomata induced by incomplete Freund adjuvant has been achieved (Spector, Lykke and Willoughby, 1967). The procedure was to transfuse syngeneic 3HT-labelled leucocytes into rats with granulomata of various ages and then compute the number of fresh macrophages entering the lesions in the 24-hour period between the time of the transfusion and the deaths of the rats. Granulomata with high turnover of macrophages showed a sustained entry of 200,000 mononuclear cells each in twenty-four hours. In carrageenan-induced granulomata with a low turnover of macrophages, the entry of circulating macrophages is, after an initial spurt, one tenth of this or less (Ryan and Spector, 1969). Comparing reactions to carrageenan on the one hand and to Freund adjuvant on the other, it is apparent that rates of sustained macrophage emigration and proliferation proceed in parallel.

Recent work (Ryan and Spector, 1970) has established the relationship between recruitment and proliferation of macrophages more clearly. Studies have shown that, in granulomata induced by injection of *B. pertussis* vaccine, there is a very high turnover of macrophages, owing, presumably, to some toxic effect of the inoculum on the cells. In rats with granulomata of this type, even lesions present for a long time, destruction of the bone marrow with shielding of the reaction site is followed within twenty-four hours by virtual cessation of DNA synthesis in the granuloma macrophages. Similarly, macrophages teased out of such lesions in nonirradiated animals show no DNA synthesis, although the corresponding rate in the macrophages seen in sections of the lesion itself is high. These results show that, even in six-week-old granulomata due to *B. pertussis* vaccine, most of the macrophages are very recent arrivals from the bone marrow and have a high rate of proliferation.

The results for the carrageenan-induced granuloma, in which there is a low turnover of macrophages, are in complete contrast to those for the *B. pertussis*-induced reaction (Ryan and Spector, 1969; Spector and Ryan, 1969). In rats with one-week-old carrageenan-induced lesions, destruction of the marrow by X-ray irradiation causes only a moderate fall in the DNA-synthesis rate of macrophages in the lesions; and, in mature reactions to carrageenan (i.e. in reactions of six weeks' duration or so), destruction of the bone marrow by X rays leads to no fall at all in the already low DNA-synthesis rate in the macrophages of the lesion. On the other hand, irradiation of the reaction site results in total cessation of such DNA synthesis as is demonstrable in the macrophages. Similarly, macrophages teased out of mature carrageenan lesions show a level of DNA synthesis as high as that seen in the parent reaction. These results demonstrate the existence of a granuloma in which recently arrived perivascular macrophages are virtually absent. The major significance of this experiment, however, lies in its demonstration that, by virtue of both longevity and mitotic division, macrophages can develop into a population independent of fresh recruitment.

All these results indicate that DNA-synthesizing inflammatory macrophages fall into three classes—recent arrivals from the circulation, members of a population heavily dependent on constant recruitment from the marrow, and members of a self-sufficient local population largely independent of such recruitment.

The macrophages of reactions to *B. pertussis* vaccine are mainly in the first group; those of glass-coverslip reactions are mainly in the second group; and those of carrageenan-induced granulomata are mainly in the last group.

The direct relationship between the extent of sustained macrophage immigration and the amount of macrophage proliferation is most simply explained by the hypothesis that both sources of cell replenishment are stimulated by the release of factors resulting from damage to the granuloma macrophages.

Such damage could well be brought about by ingestion of cytotoxic irritant; the system as a whole would then constitute a homeostatic mechanism which, by keeping up the numbers of available macrophages, would prevent the systemic release of free irritant. The nature of such hypothetical mitogenic and chemotactic factors remains purely speculative. There is, however, some evidence to show that specific chemotaxis of monocytes may occur (Ward, 1968; Wilkinson *et al.*, 1969) as a result of activation of specific serum components by many mechanisms, including substances released from damaged macrophages.

It is obvious from all that has gone before that the three mechanisms for maintaining macrophage population in a chronic inflammatory situation i.e. proliferation, longevitiy, and recruitment from circulating cells) are demonstrable in different degrees in differing types of inflammation. Two main types of chronic inflammation seem to exist—those involving high macrophage turnover and those involving low macrophage turnover. The former relies mainly on macrophage proliferation and recruitment, the latter mainly on macrophage longevity. With the passage of time, proliferation and recruitment of macrophages tend to be replaced by cell longevity, owing perhaps to natural selection amongst the macrophage population or to loss of toxicity by the irritant.

A further difference between granulomata with high turnover of macrophages and those with low turnover is the pattern of distribution of irritant. In the former, as induced by ^{125}I-labelled *B. pertussis* vaccine, there is an initial period in which the particles are present in almost all macrophages of the lesion; a very prolonged period follows in which a relatively small number of central macrophages containing irritant are surrounded by a mass of irritant-free cells. Eventually, these peripheral cells disappear, leaving the central core of organism-laden macrophages, many of which, as we have seen, are of the long-lived variety. On the other hand, in granulomata with low macrophage turnover, such as granulomata provoked by carrageenan, the irritant is early demonstrable in almost all the macrophages and remains so distributed throughout the life

of the reaction. In lesions due to paraffin oil, in which macrophage turnover evolves from high to low, the irritant is, at first,
present in only some of the participating cells but is, in the
final stages of the reaction, demonstrable in all the cells present (Ryan and Spector, 1969).

Macrophages in Pneumonia

When granulomatous pneumonia is induced by endotra-
cheal injection of appropriate irritants, such as BCG or carrageenan, substantial segments of the lung become consoli-
dated, owing to infiltration by macrophages. By use of the
techniques described above, it has been shown that these cells,
like their connective-tissue counterparts, are derived from circulating monocytes of bone-marrow origin. Alveolar macrophages differ from similar cells elsewhere in a number of
ways—for example, in their respiratory patterns. In inflammation, their main peculiarity is their persistence in dividing
and maturing within the lung before being expelled into the
alveolar space (Velo and Spector, 1973). This process of
expulsion may be detected by collecting the cells by tracheal
lavage. The process reveals the efficiency with which the ex-
port of intracellular irritant is conducted. There are, however,
always some irritant-containing macrophages left in the lung,
and these exhibit the characteristics of one or the other of the
two general kinds of granulomata, depending on the stimulus
(e.g. BCG or carrageenan, as seen in subcutaneous tissue). It
seems very likely that it is these nidi of immobilized macrophages that lead to the fibrosis characteristic of many chronic
pulmonary granulomata.

The Cause of Persistent Infiltration by
Inflammatory Macrophages

Persistent infiltration by macrophages in inflammation is
synonymous with chronicity. The authors' studies at this writing indicate that failure to digest phagocytosed irritant completely is the essential common factor in chronicity. The injection of molecular aggregates or particles of various types,
labelled with ^{125}I, followed by autoradiographic study of their

fate in living tissues has shown that persistence of irritant within macrophages is invariably accompanied by persistent collections of such macrophages, whereas removal of irritant leads to disappearance of macrophages (Ryan and Spector, 1970; Spector and Heesom, 1969; Spector, Heesom and Stevens, 1968). Comparing the disintegration by macrophages of granuloma-inducing and nongranuloma-inducing organisms (e.g. *B. pertussis* and *Staphylococcus albus*, respectively) shows that, at first, both types of particles are rapidly degraded to soluble products *in vivo* and *in vitro*, but that, whereas with the staphylococcus, degradation proceeds to completeness, the breakdown of granulogenic organisms virtually ceases about the fourth day, when some 10 percent of the original radioactivity is still attached to insoluble organisms or fragments of organisms.

Failure of inflammatory macrophages to digest foreign material such as talc, carbon, or carrageenan, is easy to understand, since either such material is inherently nondegradable or the macrophages lack the enzymes required for its hydrolysis. On the other hand, a similar failure to degrade bacteria or insoluble antigen-antibody complexes (Spector and Heesom, 1969), presents a problem; for the macrophage is well endowed with enzymes capable of breaking down complex molecules composed of naturally occurring chemical groupings. This is borne out by the observations cited above of the initially rapid degradation of granulogenic particles. The explanation of these observations is a matter for conjecture; but it may be that, after a certain period within macrophages, the ingested particles for some reason become resistant to digestion and then act as a stimulus to granuloma formation.

The relationship of hypersensitivity to chronic inflammation is complex. There may be a link between the hypersensitivity granuloma described by Epstein (1967) and the "high-turnover" granuloma described above, especially if hypersensitivity to the irritant or to an endogenous antigen can itself cause macrophage proliferation and emigration. Sensitization can convert a local reaction to a soluble protein from acute to granulomatous form (Glynn, 1968). Such sensitization, however, leads to greatly prolonged retention of antigen; this might conceivably be due to an excess of antibody available for combination. There is evidence, however, from the work of Heilmeyer, Kasemir and Kerp (1968) and Willoughby and Ryan (1970), that interference with immunological mechanisms greatly reduces the size of granulomata induced by the implantation of cotton pellets. The results of Willoughby and Ryan suggest that innate hypersensitivity to an endogenous antigen, as suggested, for example, by Glynn (1968), may be the operative mechanism.

Epithelioid Cells

There is no dispute over the essential ultrastructural features of epithelioid cells or of their origin from macrophages. Epithelioid cells have elaborate interdigitating plasma membranes applied but not fused to their neighbors. The nucleus is elongated and there is abundant cytoplasm, containing a large Golgi apparatus, many lysosomes and mitochondria, rough endoplasmic reticulum and lipid bodies, but little or no evidence of phagolysosomes.

The authors of this chapter have succeeded in maintaining cultures of epithelioid cells derived from peritoneal macrophages or blood monocytes. Virgin macrophages develop epithelioid characteristics within a week, but macrophages which have phagocytosed indigestible material (e.g. dead tubercle bacilli) fail to do so. Epithelioid cells themselves have a life span of only about three weeks but are capable of division, each cell yielding two small round cells that resemble lymphocytes but are actually young macrophages. Epithelioid cells are poorly phagocytic but actively pinocytic, especially for large suspensoids, such as colloidal gold. The evidence suggests that they are essentially macrophages which have developed along a pathway leading to intense secretory, pinocytic, and exocytic activity at the expense of phagocytic ability (Papadimitriou and Spector, 1971).

The Macrophage and Anti-Inflammatory Drugs

A number of clues indicate that both steroidal and nonsteroidal anti-inflammatory drugs may exert their beneficial effects by virtue of an action on the macrophage and its precursors. This is true not only of the glucocorticosteroids (Thompson and van Furth, 1970) but also of such nonsteroidal drugs as indomethacin. Willoughby and his colleagues have shown that these compounds inhibit the development of inflammatory edema in direct proportion to their inhibition of monocyte infiltration. These drugs inhibit monocyte migration and produce striking ultrastructural changes in macrophages. Effects on macrophage mobility and membranes could be linked with the observed influence of the nonsteroidal anti-inflammatory drugs on the prostaglandin system (Di Rosa and Willoughby, 1971). It seems almost certain that future work will throw more light on these interrelationships.

REFERENCES

Cliff, W. J.: The behavior of macrophages labelled with colloidal carbon during normal healing in rabbit-ear chambers. *Q J Exp Physiol, 51:* 112, 1966.

Cronkite, E. P., Bond, V. P., Fliedner, T. M., and Killmann, S. V.: In Haemopoiesis, Ciba Foundation Symposium, Churchill, London, 1960, p. 70.

Di Rosa, M., and Willoughby, D. A.: Screens for anti-inflammatory drugs. *J Pharm Pharmacol, 23:* 297, 1971.

Ebert, R. H., and Florey, H. W.: The extravascular development of the monocyte observed *in vivo. Br J Exp Pathol, 20:* 342, 1939.

Epstein, W. L.: Granulomatous hypersensitivity. *Prog Allergy, 11:* 36, 1967.

Giroud, J. P., Spector, W. G., and Willoughby, D. A.: Bone-marrow and lymph-node cells in the rejection of skin allografts in mice. *Immunology, 19:* 857, 1970.

Glynn, L. E.: The chronicity of inflammation and its significance in rheumatoid arthritis. *Ann Rheum Dis, 27:* 105, 1968.

Heilmeyer, L., Kasemir, H., and Kerp, L.: Thymus and inflammation. *Ger Med Mon, 13:* 441, 1968.

Huber, H., Douglas, S. D., and Fudenberg, H. H.: The IgG receptor; an immunological marker for the characterization of mononuclear cells. *Immunology, 17:* 7, 1969.

Kosunen, T. U., Waksman, B. H., Flax, M. H., and Tihen, W. S.: Radioautographic study of cellular mechanism in delayed hypersensitivity. I. Delayed reactions to tuberculin and purified proteins in the rat and guinea pig. *Immunology, 6:* 276, 1963.

Papadimitriou, J. M., and Spector, W. G.: The origin, properties, and fate of epithelioid cells. *J Pathol, 103:* 187, 1971.

Ross, R., Everett, N. B., and Tyler, Ruth: Wound-healing and collagen formation. VI. The origin of the wound fibroblast studied in parabiosis. *J Cell Biol, 43:* 119a, 1969.

Ryan, G. B., and Spector, W. G.: Macrophage turnover in inflamed connective tissue. *Proc R Soc Lond [Biol], 175:* 269, 1970.

Ryan, G. B., and Spector, W. G.: Natural selection of long-lived macrophages in experimental granulomata. *J Pathol, 99:* 139, 1969.

Spector, W. G., and Heesom, N.: The production of granulomata by antigen/antibody complexes. *J Pathol, 98:* 31, 1969.

Spector, W. G., and Lykke, A. W. J.: The cellular evolution of inflammatory granulomata. *J Pathol Bact, 92:* 163, 1966.

Spector, W. G., and Ryan, G. B.: New evidence for the existence of long-lived macrophages. *Nature, 221:* 860, 1969.

Spector, W. G., and Willoughby, D. A.: The origin of mononuclear cells in chronic inflammation and tuberculin reactions in the rat. *J Pathol Bact, 96:* 389, 1968.

Spector, W. G., Heesom, N., and Stevens, J. E.: Factors influencing chronicity in inflammation of the rat skin. *J Pathol Bact, 96:* 203, 1968.

Spector, W. G., Lykke, A. W. J., and Willoughby, D. A.: A quantitative study of leucocyte emigration in chronic inflammatory granulomata. *J Pathol Bact, 93:* 101, 1967.

Spector, W. G., Walters, M. N-I., and Willoughby, D. A.: The origin of the mononuclear cells in inflammatory exudates induced by fibrinogen. *J Pathol Bact, 90:* 181, 1965.

Thompson, J., and van Furth, R.: The effect of glucocorticosteroids on the kinetics of mononuclear phagocytes. *J Exp Med, 131:* 429, 1970.

van Furth, R., and Cohn, Z. A.: The origin and kinetics of mononuclear phagocytes. *J Exp Med, 128:* 415, 1968.

Velo, G. P., and Spector, W. G.: The origin and turnover of alveolar macrophages in experimental pneumonia. *J Pathol, 109:* 7–19, 1973.

Volkman, A., and Gowans, J. L.: The production of macrophages in the rat. *Br J Exp Pathol, 46:* 50, 1965a.

Volkman, A., and Gowans, J. L.: The origin of macrophages from bone marrow in the rat. *Br J Exp Pathol, 46:* 62, 1965b.

Ward, P. A.: Chemotaxis of mononuclear cells. *J Exp Med, 128:* 1201, 1968.

Wilkinson, P. C., Borel, J. F., Stecher-Levin, Vera J., and Sorkin, E.: Macrophage and neutrophil-specific chemotactic factors in serum. *Nature, 222:* 244, 1969.

Willoughby, D. A., and Ryan, G. B.: Evidence for a possible endogenous antigen in chronic inflammation. *J Pathol, 101:* 233, 1970.

Chapter VI

FORMATION OF PEDAL EDEMA

IN NORMAL AND

GRANULOCYTOPENIC RATS

R. VINEGAR, A. W. MACKLIN, J. F. TRUAX,
and J. L. SELPH

INTRODUCTION

IN 1958, PAGE AND GOOD studied the temporal characteristics of the inflammation produced by the subcutaneous injection of egg white in normal and neutropenic rabbits. In normal rabbits, actively motile neutrophils infiltrated the site of irritation before any tissue edema was detected. The accumulation of neutrophils and the formation of edema fluid failed to take place in neutropenic animals. These observations led Page and Good to postulate that the edema resulted from the degradative action of neutrophils on connective tissue, possibly through enzymatic processes that produce substances increasing capillary permeability. Several years later, Weissmann and Thomas (1964) showed the enzymes released from lysosomal granules derived from neutrophils to be degradative and inflammatory when injected into the knee joint of the rabbit. This finding suggests that the postulate of Page and Good can be simplified, since the endogenous irritant responsible for producing the increase in capillary permeability may be the lysosomal enzymes of the neutrophil.

Several recent publications challenge the view that the direct or indirect participation of the neutrophil is required for the development of the acute inflammatory response. In 1968, Willoughby and Spector showed that the tissue edema

111

produced in response to thermal injury, skin burn, and intra-pleural injection of turpentine was similar in normal and agran-ulocytic rats. The investigators used an intraperitoneal regimen of the antimetabolite methotrexate to produce the agran-ulocytosis. In 1971, Di Rosa, Giroud, and Willoughby observed the development of carrageenan edema over the first six hours to be the same in normal and methotrexate-treated rats. This finding, however, was not confirmed by Vinegar, Truax and Selph (1971). These workers reported that, although the small first phase of the biphasic carrageenan edema (Vinegar, Schrei-ber, and Hugo 1969a) developed normally in methotrexate-treated rats, the large second phase was strongly curtailed. In rats treated with cytoxan and 6-MP, Van Arman, Risley, and Kling (1971) found the amount of edema formed in response to carrageenan to be a function of the number of circulating leuco-cytes. Recently, Arrigoni-Martelli and Restelli (1972) reported that nystatin edema was inhibited in the hindlimbs of metho-trexate-treated rats and that the degree of inhibition was a function of the number of leucocytes in the circulation.

At the beginning of this chapter, the importance of the time course of edema formation in drug-inhibition studies is demon-strated. This is followed by a characterization of the edema-time curves obtained in the hindlimb of the rat as a result of the subplantar injection of a wide variety of highly purified enzymes, biogenic amines, and chemical irritants. The effect of various drugs on the development of many hindlimb edemas is then given, along with the data indicating that all pharma-cologically induced hindlimb edemas can be grouped into three classes. Finally, development of edema of each class is compared in normal and severely granulocytopenic animals. From these results, an attempt is made to explain the differ-ences between the results of Page and Good and those of Willoughby and his coworkers.

EDEMA FORMATION IN THE RAT HINDLIMB

Advantages of Rat-Hindlimb Model of Inflammation

This past decade has witnessed a large increase in the num-ber of experimental studies which use the subcutaneous tissue of the rat hindlimb as the site of inflammation. In this model of inflammation, changes occurring in hindlimb volume after injection of an irritant are used as a measure of edema volume. The initial stimulus for the increased number of studies was the introduction of simple quantitative methods for measuring hindlimb volume by Van Arman and his associates (1965) and Vinegar (1968). With these techniques, repeated hindlimb-volume determinations can be made quickly and easily in normal unrestrained rats and changes in volume of several hundredths of a milliliter can be measured with an error of less than 3 percent. It is possible, therefore, to follow the time course of edema formation in individual animals and pool the results obtained from large numbers of animals (Winter, 1965). Unfortunately, use of these quantitative volumetric techniques has not appreciably reduced the wide variation in edema-time curves obtained in response to some irritants (Winter, 1965; Van Arman *et al.*, 1965; Vinegar, Schreiber, and Hugo 1969a). One procedure which may reduce some of this variation is to inject an irritant into one hindlimb and the solvent for the irritant into the other. Since right and left hindlimb volumes are the same initially, the difference in volume between the two limbs is a measure of the edema produced; and variations in hindlimb volume occurring during the course of the day as the degree of hydration of the host changes do not affect the calculated edema volumes. This procedure is used in the studies outlined in this paper but has not been widely accepted by other investigators.

Another reason for the wide use of the rat-hindlimb model of inflammation, particularly among pharmacologists, is the strong sensitivity of a few hindlimb edemas to relatively low doses of steroidal and nonsteroidal anti-inflammatory drugs. In addition, the drug selectivity of these edemas, as indicated by insensitivity to antihistaminic and antiserotonin agents (Winter, 1965; Van Arman *et al.*, 1965; Vinegar, 1968), enhances their importance as pharmacological tools. Another advantage of the hindlimb model is the ease with which a simple technique allows histological study of the hindlimb inflammation at all stages of development. The histological observations can be correlated with the quantitative measurement of hindlimb-edema volume.

Formation of Kaolin Hindlimb Edema

Hillebrecht (1954) reported that relatively low doses of some steroidal and nonsteroidal anti-inflammatory drugs inhibit the edema produced by kaolin in the hindlimb of the rat at the end of five hours. His findings were confirmed in several laboratories (Lorenz, 1961; Wagner-Jauregg, Jahn and Buech, 1962; Vinegar, 1968). When the authors of this chapter, however, and others (Frey and Rothe, 1965) studied inhibition of

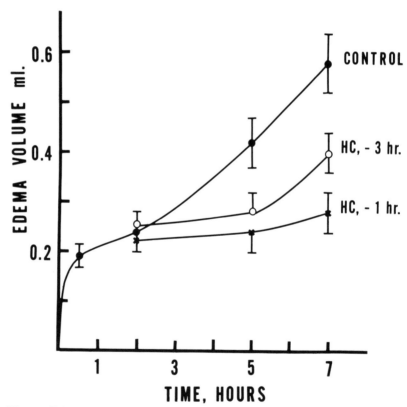

Figure VI-1. Effect of one- and three-hour pretreatment with hydrocortisone (HC, 50 mg/kg, i.p.) on the time course of kaolin-edema formation. There were six rats in each group. The edema resulting from injection of the solvent in one hindlimb has been subtracted.

kaolin edema at the end of five hours as a function of the dose of hydrocortisone or phenylbutazone, the response was found to be broad, and a quantitative measure of the potency of these drugs could not be made. A possible explanation of the broad dose-response curves became apparent several years later when the effect of hydrocortisone on kaolin edema was studied as a function of time (Figure VI-1). This adrenocorticoid did not inhibit the quantity of edema produced at the end of two hours; however, almost complete inhibition of the edema formed between the second hour and the fifth was obtained. Since the two-hour control volume was about half the five-hour control volume and hydrocortisone did not inhibit the two-hour volume, it was not possible for that drug to produce more than 50 percent inhibition of the five-hour volume. The presence of a significant component of the total edema measured at the end of five hours, a component insensitive to hydrocortisone, accounts for much of the broadness of the dose-response to hydrocortisone. Prednisolone, betamethasone, and the non-steroidal anti-inflammatory drugs, indomethacin and phenylbutazone, produce the same qualitative changes in the time course of kaolin-edema formation as hydrocortisone does. These results lead us to suggest that two distinct mechanisms are responsible for the acute edematous response to kaolin: One produces edema within the first two hours and is relatively insensitive to indomethacin, phenylbutazone, and anti-inflammatory corticosteroids; the other produces edema between the second hour and the fifth. The second mechanism is very sensitive to both steroidal and nonsteroidal anti-inflammatory agents.

Once the importance of time in the course of kaolin-edema formation was fully realized, a standard edema-time curve for kaolin could be established. This standard curve exhibited two periods of accelerated edema formation in the first seven hours and was therefore analyzed as a biphasic event (Vinegar, 1968). Four other lines of evidence support that conclusion:

1. Some anti-inflammatory drugs are able to block development of the second phase without affecting the first (Figure VI-1).

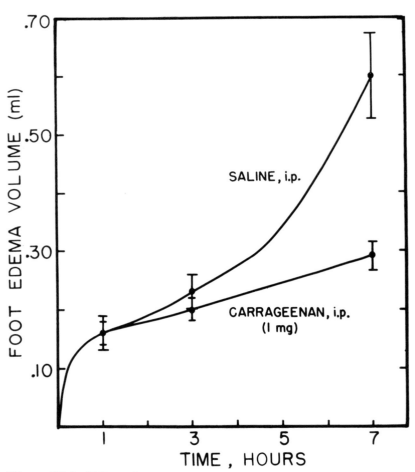

Figure VI-2. Effect of pretreatment with carrageenan or pyrogen-free saline on the time course of kaolin-edema formation. Carrageenan (1 mg, i.p.) or saline was given one hour before the kaolin. There were six rats in each group. Kaolin (5 mg) was injected into one hindlimb. The other hindlimb was injected with 0.05 ml of pyrogen-free water, the solvent for the kaolin. The edema resulting from the injection of the water has been subtracted.

2. When 0.20 mg of kaolin is injected into the hindlimb of the rat instead of the usual 5.0 mg, the full first phase develops but the second does not (Vinegar, 1968).

3. The intraperitoneal injection of an irritant one hour before the subplantar administration of 5 mg of kaolin results in strong inhibition of the second phase without any effect on the first (Figure VI-2).

4. In severely granulocytopenic rats, the first phase develops normally but the second is strongly curtailed (Figure VI-3).

As the mediators responsible for each phase of kaolin edema are still unknown, the factors determining the magnitude of their effects remain uncontrolled. In kaolin-edema research, this lack of control results (1) in great variation in ratio of magnitude between the volume of the first phase and that of the second from day to day in the same laboratory and (2) in even greater variations between the results of different investigative groups. Experience has shown that the second phase may account for 30 to 70 percent of the five-hour volume of edema. In experiments in which the second phase accounts for only 30 percent of that volume, drug inhibition of the edema will be small and no ED50 value will be induced by adrenocorticoids, indomethacin, or phenylbutazone. When the second phase accounts for 70 percent of the five-hour volume of edema, however, drug inhibition of the edema will be greater and ED50 values can be obtained. Much of this variation can be circumvented by using inhibition of the second phase for evaluating anti-inflammatory compounds (Vinegar, 1968). When this is done, changes in the magnitude of the first phase are not a factor. In addition, changes in the magnitude of the second phase are not important, for the drug sensitivity of that phase is only weakly dependent on its magnitude. Since the second phase is very sensitive to adrenocorticoids, the authors of this chapter have always been careful in the manipulation and treatment of their laboratory animals before and during an experiment. Each animal is handled the same number of times and the number of foot readings kept minimal. To obtain a

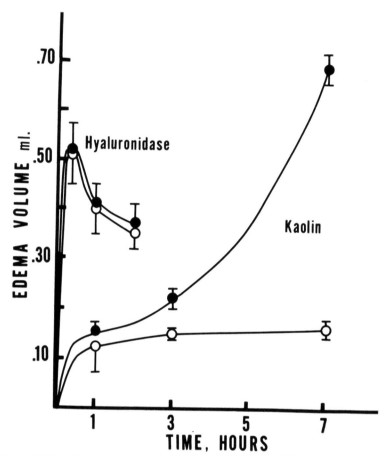

Figure VI-3. Development of kaolin and hyaluronidase edema in untreated and methotrexate-treated animals. The closed circles represent
the untreated group and the open circles the low-neutrophil, methotrexate-treated animals.

standard edema-time curve, a separate group of animals is
used for each point on the curve.

Complicating the shape of the dose-response curve for
many anti-inflammatory drugs in rat-hindlimb edema is the
additional edema inhibition produced as high drug levels are
reached and side effects become manifest. Since, in such
periods of stress, the rats used tend to conserve fluid, nonspecific inhibition of edema occurs. This nonspecific inhibition,

usually confined to 10 to 40 percent, can be detected by its
inception against the development of all hindlimb edemas at
the same dose level. Serotonin can be used to uncover nonspecific inhibition. Steroidal and nonsteroidal anti-inflammatory drugs do not inhibit the formation of serotonin edema
at dose levels which strongly curtail the second phase of the
biphasic edemas.

Formation of Carrageenan Hindlimb Edema

About the time that the importance of the biphasic nature
of kaolin-edema formation became apparent, Winter and his
colleagues (1962) introduced the carrageenan assay for anti-
inflammatory activity in the rat hindlimb. Several years later,
studies of the time course of carrageenan-edema formation
showed it to be biphasic over the first three hours (Vinegar,
Schreiber and Hugo, 1969a). Six lines of evidence now sub-
stantiate this:

1. The edema-time curve has two periods of accelerated edema
   formation (Figure VI-4).

2. Readings of hindlimb-foot-skin temperatures exhibit two hy-
   perthermic periods corresponding in time to the two periods
   of accelerated edema formation (Vinegar, Schreiber, Hugo,
   1969a).

3. Adrenocorticoids and indomethacin block the development of
   the second phase without affecting the first (Figure VI-4).

4. Subplantar injection of carrageenan heated at 130° C for six-
   teen hours results in full development of the first phase without the second.

5. Intraperitoneal administration of 1 mg of carrageenan before
   subplantar injection of carrageenan (counter-irritant action)
   results in 85 percent inhibition of the second phase without
   having any appreciable effect on the first (Vinegar and Truax,
   1970; Figure VI-5).

6. In severely granulocytopenic rats, the first phase develops
   normally but the second is strongly inhibited (Figure VI-6).

Recently, Di Rosa, Giroud and Willoughby (1971) analyzed the acute edematous response to carrageenan in the
rat hindlimb as a triphasic event over the first six hours and
subsequently reported that nonsteroidal anti-inflammatory

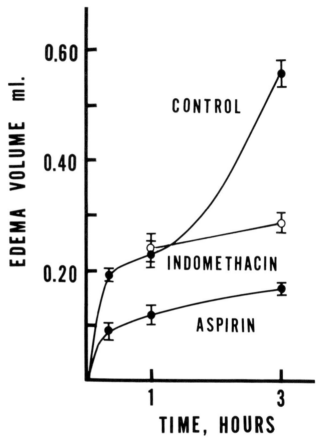

Figure VI-4. Effect of indomethacin (10 mg/kg, p.o.) and aspirin (300 mg/kg, p.o.) on the time course of carrageenan-edema formation. The drugs were given orally one hour before the carrageenan. There were six rats in each group. Carrageenan (0.5 mg) was injected into one hindlimb. The other hindlimb was injected with 0.05 ml of pyrogen-free saline, the solvent for the carrageenan. The edema resulting from injection of the saline has been subtracted.

drugs failed to influence the early development of edema (Di Rosa, Papadimitriou and Willoughby, 1971). Their triphasic analysis was based on the changes in the edema-time curve produced by various pharmacological agents. However, the shape of the curve drawn from the foot-edema data they presented was biphasic (Di Rosa, Papadimitriou and Wil-

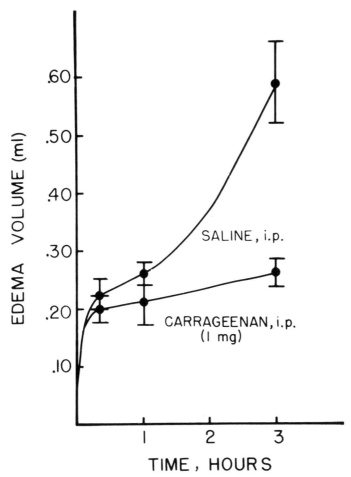

TIME , HOURS

Figure VI-5. Effect of pretreatment with carrageenan or pyrogen-free saline on the development of carrageenan edema. Carrageenan (1.0 mg, i.p.) or pyrogen-free saline was given four hours before the subplantar carrageenan. There were six rats in each group. Carrageenan (0.50 mg) was injected into one hindlimb. The other hindlimb was injected with pyrogen-free saline, the solvent for the carrageenan. The edema resulting from the injection of the saline has been subtracted.

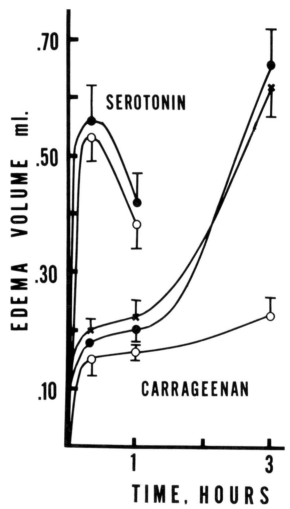

Figure VI-6. Development of serotonin and carrageenan edema in untreated and methotrexate-treated animals. The closed circles represent the untreated group and the open circles the low-neutrophil methotrexate-treated animals. The high-neutrophil methotrexate-treated group given carrageenan is represented by the symbol *x*.

loughby, 1971). The first phase was exceptionally massive and ended one-and-a-half hours after the subplantar injection of carrageenan. Most of the edema of this phase, 1.17 ml, was present at the end of one hour. This one-hour volume is five times larger than the corresponding value published by Winter (1965), Van Arman and his coworkers (1965), and Vinegar, Schreiber and Hugo (1969a) and indicates that there is a fundamental difference between the system studied by Di Rosa, Papadimitriou and Willoughby (1971) and that studied by the other investigators. Di Rosa, Giroud and Willoughby (1971) were able to delay the development of the large one-hour volume by treating their animals for four days with B.W. 48-80 or by administering cyproheptadine and the antihistaminic mepyramine to them simultaneously. After a delay of about an hour, edema production rebounded in the animals given either regimen. Hindlimb edema equal to that produced in control animals was present at the end of two-and-a-half hours. Both regimens reduced the exceptionally large one-hour volume to the small value reported by the other three groups; Di Rosa, Giroud and Willoughby (1971) and Di Rosa (1972) therefore attempted an analysis of the mediators responsible for that small one-hour volume. Such an analysis was, however, not justified. According to the data presented by Di Rosa, Papadimitriou and Willoughby (1971), the second phase of accelerated edema formation occurred between the second and the third hour, the volume of edema being 0.32 ml. All the anti-inflammatory compounds tested by Di Rosa, Papadimitriou and Willoughby (1971) produced more than 50 percent inhibition of the second phase. There was no indication, either in their own edema-time data or in the curves published by the other investigators, of a third period of accelerated edema formation.

Characteristics of Edema-Time Curves

The subplantar injection of a large number of irritants into the hindlimb of the rat has led to discovery of four distinct groups of edema-time curves. Some members of each group, as well as a few of their characteristics, are listed in Table VI-I.

TABLE VI-I

SOME CHARACTERISTICS OF VARIOUS EDEMAS IN
THE RAT HINDLIMB

Edema-Time-Curve Group	General Shape of Edema-Time Curve	Hindlimb Irritant-Solvent	µg/Limb	Time to Peak Vol. (min)
1	Rapid onset, Rapid approach to peak, Rapid decay; monophasic	Hyaluronidase-w Serotonin-s	25 2	20 20
2	Rapid onset, Rapid approach to peak, Slow decay; monophasic	Acid Phosphatase-w Elastase-w Trypsin-w Dextran-w	100 50 100 50	20 60 60 60
3	Rapid onset, Gradual approach to peak; monophasic	Lipase-w Ribonuclease-w Formalin-w	100 100 1,000	180 120 120
4	Biphasic	Collagenase-w Carrageenan-s Kaolin-w	50 500 5000	20;120 60;180 120;420

There were at least five rats in each experimental group. The abbreviations *w* and *s* represent the solvents pyrogen-free water and pyrogen-free saline, respectively. The semicolon separates the time to peak volume of the first and second phases of the biphasic edemas.

Each group involves at least one enzyme, although not all enzymes are irritants. Beta-glucuronidase, lysozyme, and lactic-acid dehydrogenase are not associated with increased foot-edema volumes.

THREE CLASSES OF PHARMACOLOGICALLY INDUCED HINDLIMB EDEMA

General Considerations

Separation of all representatives of the four groups of edema-time curves into three classes of pharmacologically induced edema (Table VI-II) was made possible by the specificity exhibited by aspirin, hydrocortisone, and cyproheptadine at the relatively low dose levels selected. The use, for example, of aspirin at the level of 100 mg/kg (i.p.) resulted from earlier studies showing that a dose of 200 mg/kg produced a minimum of 10 to 30 percent inhibition of all hindlimb edemas in the rat. In addition to the nonspecific anti-inflammatory activity, that dose reduced the body temperature of normal rats. Lowering the dose from 200 to 100 mg/kg eliminated the decrease in

TABLE VI-II

THE EFFECT OF VARIOUS DRUGS ON IRRITANT- AND
ENZYME-INDUCED EDEMA

Class of Pharma-cologically Produced Edema	Hindlimb Irritant	Percentage of Inhibition of Edema Formation		
		Aspirin 100 mg/kg. i.p.	Hydro-cortisone 50 mg/kg. i.p.	Cypro-heptadine 10 mg/kg. i.p.
1	Collagenase	7;38	22;54	29;0
	Carrageenan	13;63	4;65	0;0
	Kaolin	21;80	0;72	10;0
2	Elastase	0	0	0
	Trypsin	15	5	0
3	Hyaluronidase	0	11	97
	Serotonin	0	0	100
	Acid Phosphatase	0	0	98

The semicolon separates the % inhibition of the first and second phases of the biphasic edemas.

body temperature and the small degree of nonspecific inhibition of edema formation by such irritants as serotonin and trypsin. The second phase of the biphasic kaolin and carrageenan edemas, however, was still inhibited more than 50 percent by the low dose.

Class 1

Edemas of this class are sensitive to steroidal and nonsteroidal anti-inflammatory drugs and insensitive to antiserotonin agents (e.g. the second phase of edemas produced by carrageenan, kaolin, and collagenase). The insensitivity of the three-hour carrageenan swelling to cyproheptadine was originally reported by Winter, Risley and Nuss (1962) and confirmed by Van Arman and his associates (1965). Others have demonstrated the insensitivity of the second phase of carrageenan (Vinegar *et al.*, 1969a), kaolin (Vinegar, 1968), and collagenase edemas (Vinegar and Schreiber, 1969) to cyproheptadine.

Steroidal and nonsteroidal anti-inflammatory drugs have been shown to produce dose-dependent inhibition of the second phase of kaolin (Vinegar, 1968), carrageenan (Vinegar, Schreiber and Hugo, 1969a), and collagenase (Vinegar, Schreiber and Hugo, 1969b) edemas. The advantages of using edemas of Class 1 for anti-inflammatory screening have been stressed in a previous publication (Vinegar, Schreiber and Hugo, 1969a).

The mediator or mediators responsible for producing the second phase of such edemas remain unknown; however, several lines of evidence indicate that histamine, serotonin, and bradykinin are not involved. The reason that histamine is not thought to be involved is that the rat hindlimb is insensitive to the level of histamine that could be obtained by mast-cell-granule release in the subplantar tissue (Rowley and Benditt, 1956). In addition, at dose levels which completely inhibit the edema produced by histamine in the guinea pig's hindlimb, the antihistaminics, chlorpheniramine and triprolidine, fail to affect carrageenan-edema development. Serotonin is thought not to moderate the second phase, since antiserotonin agents that block development of edemas of Class 3 do not affect development of those of Class 1. Finally, because the quantities of bradykinin required to induce a measurable swelling in the rat hindlimb are much larger than those attained physiologically, bradykinin is not considered an important mediator of the second phase of edemas of Class 1. Furthermore, when edema is produced in the rat hindlimb by injection of a large quantity of bradykinin, steroidal and nonsteroidal anti-inflammatory drugs do not inhibit edema formation (Vinegar, Kull and Rubin, 1970). Van Arman and Nuss (1969) have added to and summarized the evidence against bradykinin as a mediator of carrageenan inflammation and adjuvant arthritis.

Willis (1969), having demonstrated that a carrageenan-edema air-bleb exudate contains more than baseline amounts of PGE_2, led Di Rosa, Giroud and Willoughby (1971) to suggest that PGE_2 may produce that portion of the edema which develops two-and-a-half to twenty-four hours after injection of the carrageenan. It is well known, however, that drug inhibition of carrageenan hindlimb edema is maximum between the first and third hours after the carrageenan injection (Fig. VI-2; also Winter, 1965). Since aspirin and indomethacin inhibit the biosynthesis of PGE_2 (Vane, 1971), the period of inhibited biosynthesis should overlap the period of drug inhibition of the edema; but this does not occur, according to the evidence cited by Di Rosa, Giroud and Willoughby (1971). It is possible that prostaglandin biosynthesis takes place earlier in the hindlimb model of inflammation than in the air-bleb model.

Class 2

Edemas of this class are defined by insensitivity to both antiserotonin and anti-inflammatory agents (e.g. trypsin, elastase, formalin, and the first phase of the biphasic edemas). In 1961, Vogel and Marek reported that formalin, trypsin, and kaolin edemas were not inhibited by antiserotonin agents. These findings were soon confirmed (Winter, 1965; Vinegar, 1968). The pro-inflammatory activity of elastase in the rat hindlimb was first reported by Bertelli (1968), but he did not study the anti-inflammatory activity of antiserotonin agents. Vinegar, Schreiber and Hugo (1969a) reported that the first phase of carrageenan edema was insensitive to cyproheptadine. Previously, Winter (1965) and Van Arman and his colleagues (1965) had found that the three-hour edema produced by carrageenan, which represents the sum of the first and the second phase, was not changed by pretreatment with cyproheptadine.

Inhibition of trypsin-edema development by anti-inflammatory drugs was studied by Domenjoz and Mörsdorf in 1965. They found that aspirin in oral doses of 500 and 750 mg/kg inhibited trypsin edema by 35 and 38 percent respectively. Since these doses are greater than one third of the LD_{50} for aspirin in rats and ten times the ED_{50} for that drug against the second-phase edema produced by carrageenan, it is not likely that the inhibition they measured was specific. Analogous criticism of early studies of drug inhibition of formalin edema was made by Winter (1965). He was not able to obtain more than 35 percent inhibition of formalin edema with doses much larger than those which produce 50 percent inhibition of carrageenan edema. A small portion of the formalin edema does seem to be associated with the release of endogenous serotonin, since the 20 percent decrease produced by cyproheptadine, a decrease Winter (1965) reported, has been confirmed in the authors' own laboratory. In view of the strong inhibition of edemas of Class 3 by cyproheptadine (70% or more, the role of serotonin in the development of formalin edema is considered of secondary importance. The first phase of the biphasic edemas is insensitive to anti-inflammatory corticoids and indomethacin and is only weakly affected by aspirin and phenylbutazone (Vinegar, 1968; Vinegar, Schreiber and Hugo, 1969a).

Although the mechanism or mechanisms responsible for the development of edemas of Class 2 are unknown, some evidence indicates that they result from direct tissue damage and involve no endogenous mediator. Most of the irritant-induced edemas in Class 2 develop in less than twenty minutes, before appreciable numbers of inflammatory cells can be mobilized. Trypsin edema, one of the members of the class, is inhibited, stoichiometrically, by the local administration of soybean inhibitor (Vinegar and Schreiber, 1969). The information given above makes it reasonable to assume that trypsin and elastase, the enzymes involved in edemas of Class 2, increase the permeability of capillaries or venules by direct action. Formalin, also productive of edemas of Class 2, may act chemically at the same locus as the enzymes. Histologic examination of subplantar tissue sections, taken one and three hours after injection of trypsin and elastase, reveals the presence of inflammatory cells and tissue edema, signifying that, as a result of the tissue damage and edema produced, there is a subsequent inflammatory reaction.

Class 3

Edemas of this class are defined by an insensitivity to steroidal and nonsteroidal anti-inflammatory drugs and a high sensitivity to antiserotonin agents. Agents causing edemas of this class are hyaluronidase, 48-80, acid phosphatase, dextran, lipase, ribonuclease B, and serotonin. The ability of antiserotonin agents to block the edemas produced by hyaluronidase, 48-80, dextran, and serotonin were reported by Rowley and Benditt in 1956 and by Vogel and Marek in 1961. Ribonuclease was shown to be a rat-hindlimb irritant by Bertelli

(1968), but he did not evaluate the sensitivity of the edema to antiserotonin agents. So far, lipase has not been described as a hindlimb irritant in the rat.

The sensitivity of edemas of Class 3 to anti-inflammatory agents is difficult to assess from a review of the literature. A good many of the previous studies were carried out with little regard for the time course of edema formation in relation to drug inhibition of edema, and often poor qualitative volumetric procedures were used. Another serious weakness of many of the early studies stemmed from the popular concept that each anti-inflammatory drug should be effective against the edema provoked by every irritant. To reinforce this concept, high drug doses had to be given, and nonspecific inhibition was added to any specific anti-inflammatory activity present (Vinegar, 1970). It was not uncommon to find doses as high as the LD_{30} (Domenjoz and Morsdorf, 1965; Bertelli, 1968). At nontoxic dose levels, as Winter showed in 1965, both steroidal and nonsteroidal anti-inflammatory drugs produce less than 20 percent inhibition of serotonin edema at doses which produce more than 50 percent inhibition of carrageenan edema. He also found the anti-inflammatory agents only weakly effective against dextran edema.

The mediator of edemas of Class 3 is presumed to be serotonin released from mast cells. By observing, microscopically, the spill of granules from these cells into the surrounding tissue, Rowley and Benditt (1956) provided direct evidence of mast-cell damage by dextran, 48-80, and hyaluronidase. Interestingly, Rowley and Benditt noted that a serotonin antagonist inhibited edema formation by the mast-cell-granule-releasing agents but did not prevent cell damage. These investigators did not suggest a role for neutrophils in the development of such edemas; and histological observations by the authors of this chapter led to the same conclusion: No significant numbers of these inflammatory cells appeared in tissue sections taken twenty minutes after injection of the above-mentioned irritants, when most edemas of Class 3 are almost fully developed. One and three hours after injection of irritants producing edemas of Class 1, however, neutrophils, as well as tissue edema, were seen in the histologic sections.

EDEMA DEVELOPMENT IN GRANULOCYTOPENIC RATS

Drug-Induced Granulocytopenia

Severe granulocytopenia was first induced in rats by a modification of the methotrexate regimen outlined by Willoughby and Spector (1968). The drug was given by gavage on Days 0, 1, 2, 4, and 6, and the pro-inflammatory stimulus injected on Day 7. This regimen lessened the chance of a rebound in the number of circulating neutrophils during the period of edema formation. However, many of the difficulties encountered with the original regimen outlined by Willoughby and Spector (1968) remain. In some experiments, too few animals become granulocytopenic; in others a large percentage of the methotrexate-treated animals do not survive the regimen or are too sick to be used. Studies using other agents to produce granulocytopenia have also proved disappointing.* Preliminary experiments with the antineoplastic agent, busulphan (Myleran® Burroughs Wellcome Company), revealed that a large number of the treated animals had peripheral neutrophil counts below $100/mm^3$ of blood. These animals gained weight during the period of therapy and seemed to be in good health, although they did exhibit a prolonged blood-clotting time. Unfortunately, since the edematous response of the busulphan-treated granulocytopenic animals to serotonin was much more severe than normal, the experiments were abandoned.

Development of Edemas of Classes 1, 2, and 3 in Granulocytopenic Rats

Normal development of edemas of Class 3 in granulocytopenic animals was not unexpected, since serotonin released from the subplantar mast cells is believed to mediate that response and the number of such cells was not diminished in methotrexate-treated animals (Table VI-III). Edemas of Class 2 also developed in the granulocytopenic rats. This finding is

---

* Editor's note: An oral dose of 100 mg/kg of cyclophosphamide given to rats daily for three days may offer promise here.

TABLE VI-III
THE EFFECT OF GRANULOCYTOPENIA ON IRRITANT- AND
ENZYME-INDUCED EDEMA

Class of Pharmacologically Produced Edema	Irritant	Percentage of Inhibition of Edema Formation
		Methotrexate 2 mg/kg. p.o. (Low Neut.)
1	Carrageenan	19;85
	Kaolin	12;94
2	Elastase	0
	Trypsin	5
3	Hyaluronidase	4
	Serotonin	2
	Acid Phosphatase	8

The semicolon separates the % inhibition of the first and second phases of the biphasic edemas.

consonant with histological observations made in rats twenty minutes after they had received injections of trypsin and elastase, irritants producing edemas of Class 2; the observations did not reveal the presence of inflammatory cells, though edemas of this class are almost fully developed in rats twenty minutes after injection of the irritants.

The development of edemas of Class 1 also proved normal in animals with more than 500 neutrophils/mm³ of blood but was strongly inhibited in methotrexate-treated animals, which had peripheral neutrophil counts below 100/mm³ of blood. (Table VI-III). The importance of obtaining low circulating-white-blood-cell counts in order to demonstrate the dependence of carrageenan-edema development on the presence of the neutrophil was also clearly demonstrated in 1971 in experiments using rats with cytoxan-induced leucopenia (Van Arman, Risley and Kling, 1971; Figure VI-7). In these experiments, the magnitude of the hindlimb edema produced by carrageenan in three hours was found to be a function of the number of circulating leucocytes. Strong inhibition of edema formation (greater than 50%) was achieved when the total peripheral white-blood-cell count was less than 1,000/mm³ and the number of neutrophils less than 200/mm³. Additional evidence supporting the role of the neutrophil in the development of edemas of Class 1 was furnished by Di Rosa, Giroud, and

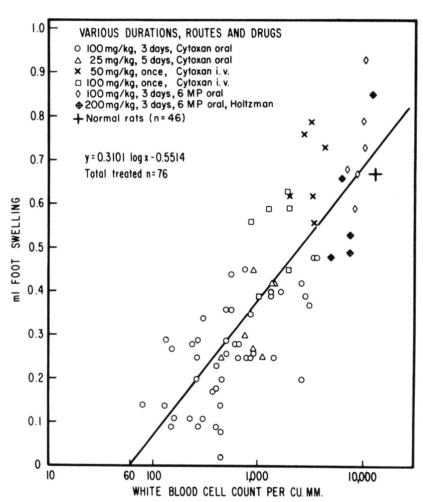

Figure VI-7. Dependence of foot swelling upon the total white-blood-cell count, showing highly significant correlation. This figure was shown by C. G. Van Arman at the meeting of the American Society for Experimental Pharmacology in Burlington, Vermont, on August 26, 1971, and is reproduced with his permission.

Willoughby, who reported that the edema formed between the first hour and the third after the injection of carrageenan (second phase) was severely curtailed in animals pretreated with antineutrophil serum. Because they obtained normal edematous responses to carrageenan in methotrexate-treated "agranulocytic" rats, Di Rosa, Giroud and Willoughby (1971) preferred to attribute the anti-inflammatory activity of the antineutrophil serum to the low titre of hemolytic complement produced by the antiserum rather than to the concomitant neutropenia. The present authors, however, as well as Van Arman, Risley and Kling (1971), have obtained strong inhibition of carrageenan edema when the peripheral neutrophil counts are severely depressed. Furthermore, the serum level of hemolytic complement does not seem to influence the development of edemas of Class 1, for animals pretreated with cobra-venom factor develop normal swellings in response to carrageenan. Cobra-venom-factor pretreatment had reduced the hemolytic level more than 91 percent. Recently, using methotrexate to produce the leucopenia, Arrigoni-Martelli and Restelli (1972) have shown a significant relationship between the number of circulating blood leucocytes and the intensity of nystatin edema in the rat hindlimb.

Several recent publications have reinforced the view that the neutrophil is important in the development of edemas of Class 1; drug inhibition of these edemas is apparently related to reduced mobilization of inflammatory cells. A recent comparative study (Van Arman *et al.*, 1971) of the subplantar tissue of untreated and indomethacin-treated rats shows that, three hours after the injection of carrageenan, an anti-edematous dose of the drug reduced the number of neutrophils mobilized. In addition, infiltration of muscle tissue by these inflammatory cells was reduced in the drug-treated group. Similar findings in aspirin-treated animals have been reported recently (Vinegar *et al.*, 1971). In untreated animals injected with carrageenan, the migration of large numbers of neutrophils into the subcutaneous tissue coincided with the formation of diffuse tissue edema of severe magnitude. A strong anti-inflammatory dose of aspirin delayed the appearance of neutrophils in the tissue and reduced the degree of tissue edema. Anti-inflammatory corticoids may act in a manner similar to the nonsteroidal just discussed, for Fruhman (1962) has shown that these steroids inhibit the intraperitoneal mobilization of neutrophils produced by endotoxin. The anti-inflammatory steroids also inhibit the pleural mobilization of neutrophils produced by kaolin (Vinegar, Truax and Selph, 1972), which produces edemas of Class 1.

In granulocytopenic rats, as the authors of this chapter have shown, the responses to irritants producing edemas of Class 2 and Class 3 are normal but the responses to irritants producing edemas of Class 1 are strongly inhibited. These findings may provide a basis for explaining some of the apparent discrepancies in the literature on the development of the acute inflammatory response in leucopenic animals (Willoughby and Giroud, 1969). Page and Good (1958), for example, found the inflammatory reaction to egg white strongly inhibited in leucopenic rabbits, whereas Willoughby and Spector (1968) reported that turpentine pleurisy and thermal skin edema develop normally in granulocytopenic rats. The irritants used by Willoughby and Spector (1968), the organic solvent turpentine and a heated brass plate with which to cause skin burns, produce direct tissue injury and elicit a rapid monophasic edematous response from the host, a response not curtailed in granulocytopenic rats (Spector and Willoughby, 1959; Willoughby and Giroud, 1969). The properties of the irritants used by Willoughby and Spector (1968) indicate that they are among those producing edemas of Class 2 or Class 3. The inflammatory reaction to egg white studied by Page and Good (1958) developed slowly. Four hours elapsed before a severe histological reaction involving inflammatory cells and tissue edema was observed. This relatively slow development, the participation of inflammatory cells, and the strong inhibition of the edema in leucopenic animals all suggest that the irritant studied by Page and Good (1958) is among those producing edemas of Class 1.

There are at least three mechanisms by which an acute edematous response can be elicited in the rat hindlimb. Two, those involved in producing edemas of Classes 2 and 3, are operative in the absence of the neutrophil; the third, involved in producing edemas of Class 1, depends on those cells. It is edemas of Class 1 that represent the "acute inflammatory response" defined and studied by the pathologist. Interestingly, it is also those edemas that are sensitive to steroidal and nonsteroidal anti-inflammatory drugs.

Complicating these rat hindlimb studies is the histological evidence indicating that an edema of Class 1 follows the development of an edema of either Class 2 or Class 3. Since these sequential reactions have not been resolved by the quantitative foot-volume measurements, it may be assumed that the component contributed by the edema of Class 1 is small. This assumpion is supported by the similarity in shape and magnitude of the time curves obtained for edemas of Classes 2 and 3 induced in normal and granulocytopenic animals.

SUMMARY

The edema-time curves produced in the rat hindlimb by a wide variety of enzymes, mediators, and chemical irritants fall into four groups. Tested for sensitivity to steroidal and nonsteroidal anti-inflammatory drugs and bioamine antagonists, edemas of these groups prove to be of three pharmacologically induced kinds: (Class 1) those highly sensitive to anti-inflammatory drugs but insensitive to antiserotonin agents, (Class 2) those relatively insensitive to anti-inflammatory drugs and antiserotonin agents; and (Class 3) those highly sensitive to antiserotonin agents but insensitive to anti-inflammatory drugs. Formation of edemas of all three classes has been studied both in normal rats and in severely neutropenic rats, with orally administered methotrexate producing the neutropenia. The results show that severely neutropenic rats (0–500 neutrophils/mm^3 of blood) develop normal edemas of Class 2 and Class 3 but not edemas of Class 1. This indicates (1) that edemas sensitive to anti-inflammatory drugs fail to develop in severely neutropenic rats and (2) that edemas not affected by those drugs develop normally in such rats.

136   *White Cells in Inflammation*

REFERENCES

Arrigoni-Martelli, E., and Restelli, A.: Development of nystatin edema and lysosomal-enzyme release at the site of inflammation in normal and leucopenic rats. Volunteer Abstract of the Fifth International Congress on Pharmacology in San Francisco, California, 1972, p. 10.

Bertelli, A.: Proteases and antiproteasic substances in the inflammatory response. *Biochem Pharmacol Suppl, 17:* 229–240, 1968.

Di Rosa, M.: Biological properties of carrageenan. *J Pharm Pharmacol, 24:* 89–102, 1972.

Di Rosa, M., Giroud, J. P., and Willoughby, D. A.: Studies of the mediators of the acute inflammatory response induced in rats in different sites by carrageenan and turpentine. *J Pathol, 104:* 15–29, 1971.

Di Rosa, M., Papadimitriou, J. M., and Willoughby, D. A.: A histopathological and pharmacological analysis of the mode of action of nonsteroidal anti-inflammatory drugs. *J Pathol, 105:* 239–256, 1971.

Domenjoz, R., and Mörsdorf, K.: Rat-paw edema induced by proteolytic enzymes as a test for the evaluation of anti-inflammatory agents. In Garattini, S., and Dukes, M. N. G. (Eds.): *Nonsteroidal and Anti-Inflammatory Drugs.* Amsterdam, Excerpta Medica Foundation, International Congress, Series N.82, 1965, pp. 162–173.

Frey, H. H., and Rothe, O.: Beitrag zur Auswertung antiphlogistischer Versuchsergebnisse. *Arzneimittel-Forsch, 15:* 92–94, 1965.

Fruhman, G. J.: Adrenal steroids and neutrophil mobilization. *Blood, 20:* 355–363, 1962.

Hillebrecht, J.: Zur routinemässigen Prüfung antiphlogistischer Substanzen in Rattenpfotentest. *Arzneimittel-Forsch, 4:* 607–614, 1954.

Lorenz, D.: Die Wirkung von Phenylbutazon auf das Pfotenödem der Ratte nach oraler Applikation. *Arch Exp Pathol Pharmakol, 241:* 516–517, 1961.

Page, A. R., and Good, R. A.: A clinical and experimental study of the function of neutrophils in the inflammatory response. *Am J Pathol, 34:* 645–656, 1958.

Rowley, D. A., and Benditt, E. P.: 5-Hydroxytryptamine and histamine as mediators of the vascular injury produced by agents which damage mast cells in rats. *J Exp Med, 103:* 399–411, 1956.

Spector, W. G., and Willoughby, D. A.: Experimental suppression of the acute inflammatory changes of thermal injury. *J Pathol Bact, 78:* 121–132, 1959.

Van Arman, C. G., and Nuss, G. W.: Plasma bradykininogen levels in adjuvant arthritis and carrageenan inflammation. *J Pathol, 99:* 245–250, 1969.

Van Arman, C. G., Begany, A. J., Miller, L. M., and Pless, H. H.: Some details of the inflammations caused by yeast and carrageenan. *J Pharmacol Exp Ther, 150:* 328–334, 1965.

Van Arman, C. G., Bokelman, D. L., Risley, E. A., and Nuss, G. W.: Changes in the rat's foot with carrageenan inflammation and indomethacin treatment. *Fed Proc, 30:* 386, 1971.

Van Arman, C. G., Risley, E. A., and Kling, P. J.: Correlation between white-cell count and inflammatory swelling induced by carrageenan in the rat's foot. *The Pharmacologist, 13:* 284, 1971.

Vane, J. R.: Inhibition of prostaglandin synthesis as a mechanism of action for aspirin-like drugs. *Nature [New Biol], 231:* 232–235, 1971.

Vinegar, R.: Chairman's report of discussion group of inflammatory processes. In Eigenmann, R. (Ed.): Proceedings of the Fourth International Congress on Pharmacology. Basel, Switzerland, Schwabe, 1970, vol. I, pp. 184–192.

Vinegar, R., Macklin, A. W., Truax, J. F., and Selph, J. L.: Histopathological and pharmacological study of carrageenin inflammation in the rat. *The Pharmacologist, 13:* 284, 1971.

Vinegar, R.: Quantitative studies concerning kaolin-edema formation in rats. *J Pharmacol Exp Ther, 161:* 389–395, 1968.

Vinegar, R., and Schreiber, W.: Serotonin as the principal mediator of many enzyme-induced edemas in the rat paw. *The Pharmacologist, 11:* 267, 1969.

Vinegar, R., and Truax, J. F.: Some characteristics of the anti-inflammatory activity of carrageenan in rats. *The Pharmacologist, 12:* 202, 1970.

Vinegar, R., Kull, Jr., F. C., and Rubin, N.: Pro-inflammatory activity of some enzymes and vasoactive amines in the guinea pig and rat. *Fed Proc, 29:* 420, 1970.

Vinegar, R., Schreiber, W., and Hugo, R.: Biphasic development of carrageenan edema in rats. *J Pharmacol Exp Ther, 166:* 96–103, 1969a.

Vinegar, R., Schreiber, W., and Hugo, R.: Some characteristics of enzyme-induced inflammation in the rat. *Fed Proc, 28:* 357, 1969b.

Vinegar, R., Truax, J. F., and Selph, J. L.: Pedal-edema formation in agranulocytic rats. *Fed Proc, 30:* 385, 1971.

Vinegar, R., Truax, J. F., and Selph, J. L.: Some characteristics of the pleural mobilization of neutrophils produced by kaolin. Fifth International Congress on Pharmacology. Abstracts of Volunteer Papers, 1972, p. 242.

Vogel, G., and Marek, M. L.: Uber die Hemmung verschiedener Rattonpfoten-Ödeme durch Serotonin-Antagonisten. *Arzneimittel-Forsch, 11:* 1051–1054, 1961.

138   *White Cells in Inflammation*

Wagner-Jauregg, Th., Jahn, U., and Buech, O.: Die antiphlogistische Prüfung bekannter Antirheumatica am Rattenpfoten-Kaolinödem. *Arzneimittel-Forsch, 12:* 1160–1162, 1962.

Weissmann, G., and Thomas, L.: On a mechanism of tissue damage by bacterial endotoxins. In Landay, M., and Braun, W. (Eds.): *Bacterial Endotoxins.* New Brunswick, Rutgers University Press, 1964, pp. 602–609.

Willis, A. L.: Release of histamine, kinin and prostaglandins during carrageenan-induced inflammation in the rat. In Mantegazza, P., and Horton, E. W. (Eds.): *Prostaglandins, Peptides and Amines.* London, Acad Pr, 1969, pp. 31–38.

Willoughby, D. A., and Giroud, J. P.: The role of polymorphonuclear leucocytes in acute inflammation in agranulocytic rats. *J Pathol, 98:* 53–60, 1969.

Willoughby, D. A., and Spector, W. G.: Inflammation in agranulocytotic rats. *Nature, 219:* 1258, 1968.

Winter, C. A.: Anti-inflammatory testing methods: Comparative evaluation of indomethacin and other agents. In Garattini, S., and Dukes, M. N. G. (Eds.): *Non-steroidal Anti-inflammatory Drugs.* Amsterdam, Excerpta Medica Foundation, International Congress Series No. 82, 1965, pp. 190–202.

Winter, C. A., Risley, E. A., and Nuss, G. W.: Carrageenan-induced edema in hind paw of the rat as an assay for anti-inflammatory drugs. *Proc Soc Exp Biol Med, 111:* 544–547, 1962.

AUTHOR INDEX

SUBJECT INDEX

A

Acetylcholine, 7
Acid phosphatase, 75, 124, 125, 128, 131
Adenosine diphosphate (ADP), 7
Adipose cells, 71
Adjuvant, 94, 101, 103, 126
Adoptive transfer, 81, 82, 83
Adrenaline (*see also* Epinephrine), 7
Adrenocorticoids, 117, 119
Afferent limb (*see* Host defense)
Afferent limb of immune function, 36
Agranulocytosis, 112, 133
Allograft, 95
Aluminum hydroxide, 80
Aluminum phosphate, 73
Alveolar macrophages, 106
Amylsulfatase, 75
Anamnestic responses, 86
Animal models, 31, 32, 37–38, 43
Antibody, 32, 38, 47, 48, 66, 79, 82, 87, 108
Antigen, 32, 48, 50, 62, 68, 71, 73, 78, 79, 80, 107, 108
 primary responses to, 59, 85
 secondary responses to, 59, 62, 86
Antigen-antibody, 4, 5, 71, 78, 107
Antigen-sensitized cells (*see* Memory cells)
Antihistamine drugs, 5, 6, 8
Antilymphocyte serum, 82
Anti-neutrophil serum, 133
Antitoxin, 62, 68, 82
Arteritis (*see* Vasculitis), 39
Arthritis, 15–28
 adjuvant, 126
 crystal-induced in dog, 25
 of gout, 28
 of pseudogout, 28
Arthus (*see* Vasculitis), 11, 38
Aspirin, 3, 6, 9, 10, 11, 120, 124–128, 133
Autologous phase, 38

B

B cells (*see also* Bone-marrow-derived lymphocytes, precursor cells), 73, 86, 87, 88
B. pertussis (*see also* Vaccine), 107
Bacteria, 31, 32, 54
Basement membrane, 39, 43
Basophilia, 59, 73
Basophilic cells, 73
BCG, 106
Beta-globulin, 31
Beta-glucuronidase, 124
Betamethasone, 115
Blast cells, 71
Boyden chamber, 37
Bradykinin, 126
Bromolysergic acid diethylamide, 5
Burn, skin, 112
Burn, syndrome, 11
Busulphan ("Myleran"), 130

C

C_2 deficiency, 49
C_3 deficiency, 48, 49
C_5 deficiency, 49
C_6 deficiency, 49
C_5 dysfunction, 49
Calcium pyrophosphate crystals, 18, 19, 20, 21, 22, 28
Capillary tube technique, 31
Carrageenan, 9, 101–107, 112, 116, 119–129, 131, 133
Cascade sequence, 33
Catecholamines, 7
 adrenalin, 7
Cathepsin, 75
Cationic protein, 8
Cellular aggregates, 68
Cellular rosettes, 65, 67, 79
Central nervous system, lupus erythematosus, 48
Cerebrospinal fluid (*see* Complement levels), 48
Chemotaxis, 31, 32, 36, 37, 38, 43, 47, 50, 51, 80, 105